MEMOIRS

of a

MEDICAL MAVERICK

First published in 2010 by
Liberties Press
Guinness Enterprise Centre | Taylor's Lane | Dublin 8
Tel: +353 (1) 415 1224
www.libertiespress.com | info@libertiespress.com

Distributed in the United States by
Dufour Editions | PO Box 7 | Chester Springs | Pennsylvania | 19425

and in Australia by
James Bennett Pty Limited | InBooks | 3 Narabang Way
Belrose NSW 2085

Trade enquiries to CMD BookSource
55A Spruce Avenue | Stillorgan Industrial Park
Blackrock | County Dublin
Tel: +353 (1) 294 2560 | Fax: +353 (1) 294 2564

Trade Paperback ISBN: 978-1-907593-02-4

Hardback ISBN: 978-1-907593-07-9

2 4 6 8 10 9 7 5 3 1

A CIP record for this title is available from the British Library.

Cover design by Orlaith Delaney and Ros Murphy
Internal design by Liberties Press
Printed by ScandBook

MEMOIRS

of a

MEDICAL MAVERICK

RISTEÁRD MULCAHY

LIB
ERT
IES

Contents

To my six children and my alma mater, St Vincent's University Hospital

ACKNOWLEDGEMENTS

I am grateful to Séamus Cashman, Aodán O'Hanlon, Ian Graham, my son, Richard, and my wife Louise for their advice while I was preparing my autobiography. I thank Richard for the use of his home as a retreat, and to him and my son, Hugh, for the use of their IT facilities. Jennifer Fisk was helpful during the production of the text and I would also like to thank Janet Cooke. Dan McAlister of the Irish Heart Foundation advised about the intricacies of internet publication. As always I am most grateful to the staff of the Central Statistics Office for their assistance. My daughters, Barbara and Lisa, gave me support and assistance. Louise has been constant in her patience and encouragement. I am grateful to Seán O'Keeffe, Daniel Bolger, Peter O'Connell, Caroline Lambe and Orlaith Delaney of Liberties Press for their roles in bringing this autobiography to final production.

INTRODUCTION

In this autobiography I write about my childhood growing up in Dublin before the Second World War; about my family, with its political and military background during the revolutionary years; about my years in the university during the war; about Aileen and my six children, and my second wife, Louise; my experience of ageing and of more than twenty years of productive retirement.

I write too about my career in medicine. I played an unusual role in my profession as a physician caring for large numbers of heart patients, as a medical epidemiologist on the international circuit researching the causes of heart disease, and as an active exponent of public health promotion and disease prevention in Ireland. Traditionally, the emphasis in medical training in the western world is on patient care; almost all practising doctors confine themselves to treating the sick or enter investigative medicine such as radiology or pathology. Few will add epidemiology, the study of disease in populations, to their clinical and research work and fewer still will add a commitment to an active public health campaign.

It is the medical epidemiologists who can best identify the causes of the common chronic diseases such as stroke, heart and respiratory disease, and cancer. Without knowledge of causes it is not possible to control these conditions or to treat them comprehensively. Identifying causes made a major contribution to reversing the coronary epidemic which arrived so unexpectedly in the mid-twentieth century. It is understandable that practising doctors in the western world are reluctant to adopt a role in public health education because of their clinical training aimed almost solely at treating the sick and their sensitivity to the charge of advertising. There is also a thin living to be earned through public health advocacy, and unfamiliarity with epidemiological research must obviously limit their understanding of the natural history of disease.

I critically examine aspects of modern medical practice and the fundamental reasons why health services in the western world seem to be in lasting crisis. I describe my close relations with the profession in Northern Ireland and in Britain, and my pride in Anglo-Irish medicine. Although my adoption of a career in medicine was more by accident than design, it proved for me to be an absorbing and exciting career, full of challenge and of the personal satisfaction which can only be derived from a close interest in the living world, and a compassion for and curiosity about humanity and Gaia, our planet home.

In latter years I have had a growing concern about the effects of the burgeoning human population, globalisation economics and waste on the imbalance between humanity and our natural surroundings, a concern which I deal with in the last paragraphs of the book. I write this account of my life and medical career at exciting and ominous times when the centuries-long deterioration in the balance between the human race and its environment is facing our children with an unpredictable and challenging future.

1

EARLY DAYS AND FAMILY
1922–1939

My father came to prominence during the Rising in 1916 when he played a crucial role in defeating a large company of armed police at Ashbourne in North County Dublin. It was the first guerrilla action during the Independence movement and guerrilla tactics were to make it impossible for the British administration and the constabulary to function in many parts of the country during the subsequent War of Independence. He was among the group of leaders which reorganised the Irish Volunteers in 1917 after the Rising and following their release from prison. He was appointed commandant of the Dublin Brigade of the Irish Volunteers shortly after his return and chief of staff of the revolutionary army during the entire War of Independence and subsequent Civil War. He was minister for defence in the early years of the State and later both minister for local government and public health and minister for education.

As children, we were always conscious of my father's reputation and of the high regard in which he was held by the people in the local community. To them I was Dick Mulcahy's son. Despite his unusual organisational abilities and his boundless energy he never attempted to seek a career in business or the professional world. He lacked personal ambition to an extraordinary degree and devoted his entire later life to his political party and his parliamentary responsibilities. It is said that the true revolutionary is one who succeeds in achieving freedom and who subsequently devotes his life to the well-being of his country.

My paternal grandfather had been postmaster in Thurles in County Tipperary. There was a strong emphasis on religion, education and the Victorian virtues of hard work and self-reliance in his family, and a tradition of conservative nationalism. The father disapproved at first of his son's Volunteer activities and his participation in the 1916 rebellion, stating that he owed much to the Westminster government for his appointment as postmaster. My grandfather lived at a time when the great majority of the people of Ireland, with the exception of the four north-eastern counties, were satisfied to achieve limited home rule and to remain within the jurisdiction of Westminster, although this was to change to a greater degree of separatism after 1916.

My father had five sisters and two brothers. Four of his sisters became teachers; three of them joined the Ursuline teaching order. The fifth remained to look after the remnants of the family after her mother's early death but then joined the Sisters of Charity. The three boys were encouraged to leave home at the age of sixteen and fend for themselves. My father's brother, Patrick, who fought in the trenches from 1915 to 1918 as a sapper in the British army, joined the Irish Volunteers after the armistice. My father's youngest brother, Sam, joined the Cistercian Order as a priest, and as abbot of the community he established the first post-Reformation Cistercian monastery in Scotland, in Presbyterian-dominated Mid-Lothian. With Presbyterians and other denominations, he led an active ecumenical movement in Scotland. His monastery was greatly welcomed by the largely Protestant Scottish population.

My father, aged twenty-one, arrived in Dublin as a post office clerk in 1907. Later, after some years of study, he qualified as a post office engineer. He joined the secret revolutionary body, the Irish Republican Brotherhood and later the Irish Volunteers, studied French and French literature and poetry, and learned both Pitman and Gregg shorthand; for the rest of his days he wrote in a mixture of both. All his life he was interested in self-education, the Irish language (which he spoke fluently) and Irish culture. His nationalist philosophy was based on cultural as much as political considerations, on Ireland's wish to control its own affairs. At all times he insisted that the army's role was to serve parliament and the people. He was satisfied that the Anglo-Irish Treaty of 1922 provided all the elements of freedom that he espoused and he had little concern about retaining the Crown and its purely symbolic connotation. He had no quarrel with the English people; his concern was with the rump of Tories who consistently opposed self-government for the Irish and who were responsible for the division of the country.

He was devoted to the Roman Catholic Church and its ministry and to the Church's great contribution to education, the social services and the national cause during and after the nineteenth century. As a leader he was forthright and decisive. During the Civil War he and his army council met in Portobello Barracks in Dublin at seven o'clock every morning. His first words in council were 'Decisions, decisions, decisions!' In the army he was regarded as a strict disciplinarian although adhering to the same precepts he expected from his men. He obviously had outstanding organisational skills, as is evident from his leadership of the army and his subsequent career as a politician and as a cabinet minister. This was also the public's perception of him.

However, his private persona was entirely different from the public perception. At the time of his death he was rightly described as affable, gracious and thoughtful of others, and that is how I remember him. He and my mother were a happy pair and the hundreds of letters between them, which are in the family archives, testify to my father's passionate nature and to my mother's ready response to his affections. Neither can I recall anything but normal and amicable relations between my brothers and sisters and myself.

Despite his being firm and decisive as a leader, as a subordinate in political life he was loyal and slow to criticise, even when policies conflicted with his own views. He never questioned the authority of his superiors. It was this characteristic which overshadowed his radicalism as a military leaders and which militated against his reputation during his later political career. By nature he was happiest when serving others and when in cabinet he tended to detach himself from the wider political scene and to devote his entire time to running his own department. In my view, his role in recent Irish history was overshadowed by his lack of personal ambition and his tendency to defer to others. I write as I do about my father because I was to realise later in life that I, and indeed my own six children, share some of his characteristics. I owe more than a little of my professional life to his example; however, I certainly never shared his degree of self-abnegation.

My father's biography, *Portrait of a Revolutionary*, was written by Maryann Valiulis in 1992 and my own memoirs about him and the family, *Richard Mulcahy: A Family Memoir*, was published in 1999; a more personal biography, *My Father, the General*, was published by me in 2009. His family had emerged from famine times and, like many Catholics who were entering the lower ranks of local and national administration towards the end of the nineteenth century, he had the advantage of the splendid education being provided by the various religious communities in nineteenth-century Ireland. This education was to bring the Catholic majority to the forefront of leadership in Ireland.

My mother's family, the Ryans, born on the family farm in County Wexford, also profited by their parents' commitment to a full and liberal education for their children. My mother's maiden name was Mary Josephine Ryan; she was invariably called 'Min' by her family and friends. She must have lived many anxious moments while my father was a fugitive from the British forces during the War of Independence and subsequently a likely recipient of an assassin's bullet during and after the Civil War. It was at a time when she was saddled with a young family and, later, estranged from some of her republican sisters after the Treaty settlement. She shared all his frustrations and anxieties with his impossible task of trying to please everybody as head of the army during the War of Independence, the prolonged truce, the immediate post-Treaty period, and the Civil War and its aftermath of demobilisation, mutiny, political division and severe economic recession.

My mother's sister, Agnes, was married to Dennis McCullough, who had been president of the separatist revolutionary Irish Republican Brotherhood before the Rising. Her eldest sister, Kate, married Sean T. O'Kelly, who was an early and prominent member of Sinn Féin and who opposed the Anglo-Irish Treaty. Later, he became a long-standing member of the Fianna Fáil cabinets up to his election as president of Ireland from 1944 to 1958. Kate died in 1934 and O'Kelly subsequently married her younger sister, Phyllis, who survived him. My mother's brother, Jim, also took part in the Rising. He opposed the Treaty and joined the inner circle of the Fianna Fáil Party, where he was a minister in its administrations, with only two three-year breaks, from 1932 until 1961. Other members of the Ryan family were active in local politics in Wexford.

Of the twelve Ryan children, eleven had a third-level education and six of the eight girls who qualified as teachers travelled to Britain and to various countries in Europe before the Great War to teach English in their religious schools. After the 1898 centenary celebrations of the 1798 rebellion, the Ryans adopted a more active form of nationalism but the 1916 Rising was to increase their sense of political radicalism and eventually to lead most of them to oppose the Anglo-Irish Treaty which ignited the Civil War, the 'compound disaster' of my father's memoirs.

From the early 1960s I began to take a keen interest in my father's career and in the recent revolutionary period. During his active career he avoided all discussion about the recent past because of the contentious issues which surrounded the Civil War and its aftermath. When he retired in 1961, I encouraged him to archive his extensive War of Independence, Civil War and political papers. Mole-like, he had retained every paper and document during his military and political career, except for his earlier War of Independence papers, which were captured by British forces in November 1920. I provided him with a secretary and with typing and recording equipment, and he threw himself with characteristic energy into the task. He spent much of his ten-year retirement in archiving his papers, in writing and in recording his many conversations with family, friends, writers, students and historians. He retained nearly all the army papers from the end of 1919 to 1924 which survived during the War of Independence, the Civil War and its aftermath. They were not released until 1971, when they were gifted to the archives of University College Dublin. They were a huge boost to these archives and are now widely used by historians and students. Their late release and delayed availability account for the fact that his seminal role as leader of the army during the entire revolutionary period was overshadowed by Michael Collins and that the many histories of Collins largely ignored the role of the General Headquarters Staff.

It was against the background of my father's history and my mother's large family that I was brought up with my three sisters and two brothers in our large, rambling house contiguous to Portobello Barracks – Lissenfield House. It was in this barracks that my father and the other army leaders conducted the Civil War. In the early years of the Free State we as a family were conscious of the political ferment in Ireland and particularly of the deep division caused by the Civil War within our own extended family. That tragedy was never far from our thoughts, although my parents and all their siblings on both sides of the Civil War divide never allowed the bitterness generated by the war to obtrude on their children, all of whom remained on normal, friendly terms. We were a close-knit extended family. The Civil War remained a forbidden subject in our households, at least until we had reached early adulthood.

My life in Lissenfield House has been described in some detail in the aforementioned *Richard Mulcahy: A Family Memoir*. My parents were so well known that, with an open-door policy prevailing and with cousins living close by, we had streams of visitors calling when most calls were casual and when it was not thought necessary (or possible) to provide food or drink. Unlike our present globalised and much-travelled world, during the 1930s and 1940s there was a great sense of community in our parish of Rathmines, with little contact with the outside world and little concern about international affairs. It was a time of few acquisitions and of greater innocence and security. A murder was a seven-day wonder. Robberies were virtually unknown because there was little to rob; nor can I recall any crime apart from a residue of political violence following the Civil War. With parents who suppressed all references to the Civil War, such events were rarely brought to our notice.

I never heard a quarrel between my parents. My mother could at times be a little irritable, but if my father were present he would touch her lightly on the shoulder and say 'Now, Min . . .' which would quickly calm her. I have more than 150 letters from him which, up to the end of their correspondence, continued to express his patient nature and his affection for her. On rare occasions he could be sharp with us children if we made inappropriate comments, particularly in relation to remarks of a critical nature: 'Haven't you something better to do than talking about things that do not concern you?'

The atmosphere of the house when we were young was practical, busy, unsophisticated and informal. We were not an overtly affectionate family. I cannot recall that I ever kissed my mother until later in life, when I left home and became conscious of the normal adult conventions, which I was to learn during my days in London. Religion played an important but intellectually limited part in our upbringing and there was still a residue of Victorian prudery. We attended mass every Sunday and I went to confession on Saturdays so that I could receive communion next day. I reported the same sin each time, received the same absolution, confirmed by saying the same three Hail Marys, and the same plea about purity; and I invariably promised never to commit the sin again. I left the confessional with a sense of relief bordering on elation. We had the old Mulcahy family Bible in the library, which came down through six generations, firstly on the Harris distaff Quaker side in the early eighteenth century and later as part of the Mulcahy Catholic heritage. It was never read by us. Bible reading was associated in our minds with our Protestant brethren, while we Irish Catholics were satisfied to accept the Church's authoritarian role in its interpretation.

Except for the thirteen years of my father's ministerial work, my mother seemed to be always pulling the devil by the tail. As a child and young adult, my abiding memory is of my mother's problems struggling to make ends meet as the wife of an impecunious politician. My father at no time had any inclination to improve his material or financial state or to undertake any gainful employment over and above his parliamentary and political duties; and these kept him well occupied. I know that in the late 1930s, when he had been in opposition for six or seven years, his annual income was £650. I know too that on a few occasions there were whip-rounds held among his colleagues and admirers to relieve his household debts.

It was against this background of financial stringency that my mother was obliged to budget for her family and for a staff of a cook, governess and resident gardener, and no doubt for her husband's pocket money. She managed through her prudence in spending but mainly by exploiting the resources of our two and a half acres to the full. She established a large vegetable and fruit garden, had a poultry farm of one hundred hens or more, occasionally a few noisy and unclean ducks, and she maintained one, sometimes two, milking cows in our field and the adjoining military field. Virtually all our needs were provided for by this mini-farm, apart from such essential items as meat, sugar, tea and flour for baking. All this was in an inner suburb in Portobello, within a mile of Grafton Street and St Stephen's Green. The meat was not infrequently pig's cheek, the cheapest in the market! She sold eggs to some of our neighbours and cousins, thus adding to her meagre housekeeping money. Whatever about my mother's stringent housekeeping allowance, she was an excellent manager of house and garden, having been brought up on her family's farm in Wexford; she managed to pass her gardening skills on to some of her children.

For a woman born on a farm, she was unusually innovative in developing a garden, having a special interest in roses and in an extensive rockery. She managed a greenhouse where tomatoes were her speciality in the summer and specimen chrysanthemums in the winter. The latter flourished in the heated greenhouse; they were sent to family friends as Christmas presents and were greatly appreciated.

We grew up under different circumstances from those of today. Because of the frugality and relative austerity of the times and the limited spending power of even the most affluent middle classes, strict prudence was necessary in all matters of household expenditure. Equipment and other household items were maintained or repaired while clothes were mostly designed and made at home, with many items passing from sibling to younger sibling. Nothing was disposed of until it was no longer serviceable; nothing was wasted. Our lives were in contrast with today's appalling waste in the western world and its certain disastrous effect on nature and the future of humanity.

Family expenses must have been small in those days. Staffs were glad of employment at salaries as low as ten shillings a week. Living with a family and becoming part of a household, with the added security of tenure, was more important to them than matters of material gain and acquisition. We lacked the materialistic preoccupations which are so evident and so destructive in today's society and we could depend on the integrity of our politicians, police and public services.

It was a more silent world and it was dark enough in the city at night to see the stars. I recall the light motor traffic, the residue of the horse-drawn vehicles. Rush hour was heralded by the horde of bicycles, undisciplined pedestrians and a degree of chaos in the streets, with a policeman on point duty at rush hour at major intersections in the city centre. Some of these men became well-known and popular figures. It was before organised traffic, so that the military bands, brass and pipe, frequently marched into the city centre and provided a disciplined and colourful spectacle in an otherwise drab and sometimes chaotic city. The military school of music, based at Portobello, was a source of pride to my family because of my father's initiative in establishing the school during the Civil War.

From 1922 to about 1934 my father had a military guard which occupied a large galvanised hut close to the avenue leading to the house. They were equipped with sub-machine guns but the weapons were only required once during the Civil War, when the house was attacked and one of the assailants, a medical student in the nearby university, was killed. The other assailants, amounting to about eighteen Irregulars, escaped through the grounds of the local church. I had just been born and I knew nothing of the affair until many years later when I read an account of the affray in a provincial paper. Yet as soon as my father resigned from the ministry of defence in 1924 he left the guard at home and travelled the four corners of Ireland without car, guard or weapon and, as he recalled, he 'never got a slap in the face'.

It is difficult to believe that we seemed to enjoy our leisure times in the 1930s without television or radio and with little cinema. The gramophone played 78 rpm records, which were mostly Moore's Melodies, and the singers always seemed to be in a hurry, no doubt because the renderings seldom exceeded two minutes. The first head of the army school of music, Colonel Fritz Brasé, one of the late Kaiser's bandmasters, composed the 'General Mulcahy March' in 1923. We had it on a 78 rpm record. It was a remarkably fast march and we always thought it was more suitable for a run!

We enjoyed indoor games and had opportunities to play tennis and to enjoy croquet on a poor grass court in summer and hurling in the adjoining military field at other times. The bicycle was our means of transport and we took the 14 or 15 tram for occasional trips to the city. We were unaware of the virtues of physical fitness and training, although some of the girls' schools taught deportment and dancing, and my parents walked at weekends or into town. Meccano and the Hornby trains were luxuries for us boys in our early teens, and stamp collecting and cigarette card collections were very much in vogue.

Scouting brought us into close contact with the boys of other families and, whatever class distinction existed within the parish, none existed among the Scouts. We were members of the Catholic Boy Scouts of Ireland, a denominational movement organised by the Catholic Hierarchy to discourage Catholic boys from joining the non-denominational Baden Powells. (Happily, both organisations have now joined as one non-denominational group.) Despite variations of affluence in the area, from the relatively well-off to the destitute, there was a natural mutual respect and courtesy among the people. Living as we were in a commodious house with extensive grounds and with my father's military and political background, my parents were treated with special consideration.

Most of the Catholics in Rathmines were first-generation families who had arrived from the provinces, and had not yet shown the urban tendency to form cliques based on affluence. However, we were only too conscious of snobbery which existed in other more affluent suburbs like nearby Donnybrook and Ballsbridge (now called 'leafy suburbs' by the media), where the more settled Catholics and Protestants, who had been educated in private boarding and day schools and were members of the more elitist tennis clubs, lived.

Scouting brought us camping in the Dublin Hills at weekends and further for our annual camps in Wexford. It knocked some of the grand ideas out of the heads of my brothers and I, which might have been generated by our relatively privileged standing in the community. It taught me many things about life and social integration which stood to me well in my later days and in my profession. It taught the value of occasional hardship and the satisfaction to be derived from service to others; it contributed to a lifetime spirit of egalitarianism and it stimulated in me an interest in nature – in trees, astronomy, geography and the countryside.

The Christian Brothers in Coláiste Mhuire, an Irish-speaking school established in 1927 by my father and his fellow cabinet minister, Ernest Blythe, provided my secondary education from 1933 to 1939. I then entered University College Dublin as a medical student. It was only in later years that I began to understand that I shared some of father's characteristics, particularly in terms of organisational skills and an inherent interest in politics and issues beyond one's own personal and professional affairs. However, I was fortunate to be spared a life in politics by entering the medical faculty whilst I was still too immature in confidence and in education to enter politics. It was only in later years, when I was established as a consultant physician in Dublin, that my wider political interests emerged through my contributions to the Irish health service, through my long association with the Irish Medical Association and my increasing involvement in medical epidemiology and health promotion.

My schooling through Irish by the Christian Brothers placed the primary emphasis on the spoken Irish language and on the Gaelic games of football and hurling. In retrospect, I thought the standard of education was poor, particularly in languages such as Latin and French. English was better because of having a good teacher. To enter the medical faculty it was necessary for me to pass Latin in the Leaving Certificate. I did so by only one mark in the pass Latin category. I headed the class in doing so and I attributed my rather doubtful distinction to having had a special grind in Latin arranged by my perceptive mother before the entrance examination.

We were not a great reading family and in my Irish-speaking school we were introduced to little English or Irish literature, drama or poetry. The only English school text I remember is *Blackcock Feather*. My earlier limited home reading was of the books based on folklore, fairy stories, legends and early Celtic mythology by the authors of the Celtic Revival: Standish O'Grady, James Stephens and, later, Padraig Colum. *The King of Ireland's Son*, *The Island of the Mighty*, *Lost on Du Corrig*, *The Coming of Cuculain*, and more than twenty other titles which are still in my home library, left me with some knowledge and consciousness of ancient Irish history and heritage. I suspect that these books, so suitable for the youth of this land, could, with greater attention by our schools and media, compete with the current Harry Potters and other recent children's bestsellers. I also have in my library the Irish-language account of our Celtic past, *An Fianna*, which was part of our school curriculum; but my memory of it is scanty, perhaps because of my neglect of the Irish language after leaving school.

I was fortunate that, having suffered an injury to my knee during my penultimate year in school, I was confined to the house for twelve weeks.

In the absence of any other occupation I started to delve through my father's library, which first stimulated my interest in biography and in Irish and natural history. My first real contact with serious reading was to lead later to the numerous sixpenny paperback Penguins, Pelicans and Penguin Classics which were popularised by Penguin Books during and after the war. Between my family and me, we have retained about six hundred copies of these old paperbacks. This collection is a virtual cornucopia of literature, science, fiction, natural history, recreation, adventure, the arts, history, biography and more which brought good quality reading at an affordable price to the masses for the first time. After a game of golf today we now talk politics, sport or the state of the stock exchange or the world; in the 1940s and 1950s we talked about our reading – and much of this was thanks to the new paperbacks. I believe that my twelve weeks away from school and my first contact with my father's library was at least as important in furthering my education as my six years in secondary school. It was a lucky break!

During my childhood and adolescence in Lissenfield no aspect of people's more intimate behaviour was ever discussed; nor, indeed, was it often in our minds. My knowledge of the mysteries of sex and of procreation was only belatedly acquired. I did not have the advantage of learning from my peers at school, as most boys did, because of the limitations of Irish, our spoken language there. Irish, at least for us children, lacked the vocabulary to delve into such an arcane subject. In terms of innocence and unworldliness, we were in striking contrast to the children we meet in schools and colleges today.

I spoke of our liberal upbringing but it was certainly not so in the modern sense of personal behaviour and morality. It was a time which differed remarkably from the mores and personal freedom of globalised culture. We were little influenced by the media and had access only to literature which lacked the modern freedom of subject and expression. We were influenced by the rigid attitude of the Church on matters of sex and body culture and their sinful connotations. In conservative, Catholic Ireland it was inevitable that sexual maturity was retarded, in my own case until my late twenties.

I was further inhibited by my five years in the university rowing club, where the culture was distinctly masculine, without the sexual connotations which might be associated with such a group. I was also inhibited by my chronic poverty which made dating impossible, not only during my university years but afterwards too during my four postgraduate years in London. I returned to Ireland a virgin and remained so for another three years. During my long years of continence I had no great urge to gratify my curiosity despite having increasing fantasies about sex; nor did I experience the strong urge for and dependence on sex which was to occur later in my life. From my initial misogyny I was to become dependent on love and on sharing my life, my joys and sorrows, and my most intimate association with another.

For some of the many priests at that time who were ordained in their early twenties the absence of sex must have been a source of loss, frustration and hardship. The Victorian attitude prevailed that sex was sinful; and irregular sexual activity was frowned upon except perhaps for the men among the upper classes – but, of course, in Catholic Ireland we had no upper class. They were innocent times. Rarely did married couples separate, and then mostly when the father emigrated to work in England or America. Many married people must have lived lives of quiet desperation.

The question of my siblings or me entering politics was never raised. My father was keen that we should have a third-level education and, now that Ireland had achieved its independence, that we should join the professions and play our parts in the normal advancement of the country's social and cultural life. With our organisational skills and work ethic, we showed some of the qualities of our parents. Both Pádraig, a quantity surveyor, and Seán, an engineer, established thriving organisations in their professional disciplines; my sister Elisabet became a scientist; my sister Máire a domestic economy instructress; and Neillí a well-known *grand couturier*.

Before I set out for London I had begun to shed my commitment to religion and the influence of the Roman Catholic Church. Clearly, one's culture can stultify one's sense of reason. Even earlier I began to question the most basic beliefs and tenets of the Church. If we were to live immortal lives in the next world, where were we before we were conceived? And was the concept of immortality so attractive? Despite the ups and downs of our lives on earth, surely this life is better than facing the meaningless immortality of the gods. Did we conceive of the idea of immortality because we are unable to conceive the world without us? I eventually became an agnostic, believing that there was a great mystery about Creation but that I was never likely to learn its nature.

Newman said that there was no point in religion if we insist on understanding all the mysteries of Creation – God, time and space, the existence of rational beings, the wonders of nature. But our very ignorance of Creation and its nature is a profound reason for recourse to spirituality. My own views are close to those of the Stoics, an elitist group formed in Greece, spreading later to the Romans before the birth of Christ and widely popularised later among the middle classes in Victorian in Britain by the *Meditations of Marcus Aurelius*. Like the Stoics, we can find a sense of spirituality by accepting virtue as a form of godliness. Our aspiration should be that virtue, like godliness, should be immanent. I may have lost my religion, but I found a new spirituality and a new comfort in the acceptance of my role as a transient but possibly purposeful entity in an unexplained universe.

In recent years I go to Sunday mass occasionally with Louise. I do so mainly to have these moments together. We walk the mile to the chapel on the campus at University College Dublin nearby. The chapel has a reasonably devotional ambience but I find the liturgy of the mass based on the goodness of God and our conviction and hope that He can put an end to the sins of mankind to be childish and unreal, as is the perceived intercessional role of Mary. There is a much greater sense of spirituality and communion with God for me when listening alone at home to Hayden's Nelson Mass or Mozart's Requiem.

As I became more concerned about my prolonged virginity and as my fantasies began to mount, I had a few minor affairs but my urges really emerged when I first met my wife, Aileen, while holidaying and golfing in Lahinch, County Clare – a Mecca of golf and of the holiday spirit. She was lively and most attractive and our relationship blossomed in a matter of a day or two. I proposed to her before leaving for home and we were married four months later. Like my parents, we had six children in rather rapid succession, a phenomenon I attributed to her remarkable fertility. We had three boys followed by three girls. And at this stage I might say that we were fortunate that our children were normal in every way; they never caused us any trouble or serious anxieties, and have been wonderfully supportive, particularly during difficult times. I am glad to detect in their traits a residue of some of their grandfather's and grandmother's genes.

I remained in love with Aileen for ten years or more; but gradually incompatibilities, some of which were initially concealed by our love, came to dominate my relationship with her. Her assertiveness was a major problem. Everything was black or white. Discussion about differences was not possible and we had little in common in terms of social, intellectual and personal matters. I suffered from depression each time I returned to the house – and instead of sharing my day with her and the children, I felt the loneliness of isolation. These incompatibilities were to increasingly affect our relationship, and I was compelled to decide that we could no longer remain together. I had an affair about five years before my departure. I was pressed to leave my family then, but I refused to do so until my eldest boy had reached his nineteenth year and had finished his schooling. After a year of solace and intimacy, mixed with guilt on my part, she departed abroad, where she found work – and a husband. She remains for me a fond memory.

Nobody, least of all my wife, was aware of my decision until the last moment before my departure from the home. My decision to leave caused considerable surprise among my friends and in my hospital. It was a most unusual event at the time for a consultant to take such drastic action and I was only too aware of the humiliation Aileen must have suffered. There was considerable pressure on me to change my mind. Two priests in particular were induced to intervene but I remained adamant. My interview with one ended in him losing his temper; the other, a close friend, was gravely disappointed but eventually had recourse to sharing a bottle of whiskey with me! The moment of parting was heart-rending. The six children were sitting in our nursery with Aileen. I simply opened the door and said goodbye. I was unable to say or do anything more. Richard accompanied me to the car. I remained mute as I got into the car. I drove away as Richard stood weeping on the gravel. I think it was the worst moment in my life.

We had two good friends in London who were particularly close to Aileen. They were generous, sociable and great company. Aileen travelled over to share her tale of woe with them and share their counsel. They phoned me and pleaded with me to visit them and Aileen in London. I replied that there was no way I would change my mind but, because of my regard for our friendship, I agreed to go over. I arrived at their flat in Kensington at about seven o'clock and the pleading started. From the start of our meeting we were being served champagne, hardly an appropriate drink for such a potentially fraught occasion. The pleading continued unabated and uninterrupted by food or other distractions, apart, that is, from the champagne; I was obdurate. We finished by becoming inebriated, maudlin, and curiously elated. I eventually fell into bed after midnight but was up early enough to catch a taxi and to board the eight o'clock plane to Dublin.

I had sought a leave of absence from the St Vincent's authorities to coincide with my departure from Lissenfield. I went immediately to France and on to Greece with my French teacher, Jacqueline Corbière. She was soon to join me as my partner for the next six years. My first month was spent on the remote Greek island of Allonisos where, strangely, my domestic troubles were entirely forgotten. We returned to France, where we stayed with her sister, Michelle, in Provence. There I wrote my first major book on the prevention of heart disease for the public, *Beat Heart Disease* (1977). Jacqueline was a *pied noir* who had come to Ireland after she and her family were pushed out of Algeria during the Algerian war. This was not her only adversity; she had many, including the loss of her parents in a car accident shortly after her arrival in Ireland.

She was a remarkably talented woman and while she was living with me she qualified from the College of Art and Design in Dublin. She was an excellent painter, designed and fabricated her own tapestries, was an accomplished linguist and teacher, sang well and played the guitar, and was an excellent cook. Despite these and other talents, our relationship proved to be unsatisfactory and incompatibilities soon emerged which finished our more intimate relationship, although she continued to live in my house for a few more years. I had become a partner of my current wife, Louise Hederman, long before Jacqueline departed my home. I eventually helped Jacqueline to buy a house and studio in Dublin and subsequently helped her to buy a house near Montpellier in France, where she now lives. We make occasional contact, usually at Christmas. We are happier together now. I treasure Jacqueline's paintings and tapestries, many of which I and my family still have hanging in our homes.

From the late 1970s I travelled the world during my years in research and as a representative of the Irish Medical Association. I was fortunate during my unsettled years to meet a kindred spirit during my travels. She was a cardiologist and a marathon runner. She shared both my intellectual and physical needs, including running every day during our meetings together. She had the firm athletic physique and the devotion to fitness which appealed most to my sensuous nature. No lovers were ever happier and more compatible. We met perhaps three or four times a year but during the intervening months between meetings I was contented by a passion in repose.

After some wonderful years it was to be a sad but inevitable separation for us when my relationship with Louise continued to blossom. We met at a meeting in France for the last time when, I intended to make the break. It so happened that our decision to end our relationship was mutual. I met her but, just as I was about to tell her of my decision, she informed me that she had fallen in love with another athlete, also a woman, who was now living with her. She regretted that her new-found friend and lover was unable to travel with her to meet me! It was an ironic end to our affair but it was a reminder of how passion often survives best during long separations. It was also a reminder that many, if not all, of us are by nature bisexual but this is so often concealed by the culture we live in.

I was always curious about the prospect of homosexual love but I had no experience in this regard nor did I ever have a wish to seek such an opportunity. However, I am capable of admiring a young and handsome athletic youth or young man, particularly seeing him with a good running style and the picture of good health, and the obvious serenity induced by well-ordered physical movement. An occasional meeting with such a person while running added to the euphoria of running. Thomas Mann, in *Death in Venice*, writes about the elderly man who spent his time on holidays following a handsome boy without making contact with him but consumed with desire for him. I could understand his dilemma. I was a dedicated runner then and I fantasised about running with a handsome young man or woman in Dublin's nature park in Sandymount on an early sunny Sunday morning, where I often ran alone in an ambience of contemplation and spiritual detachment.

What different course would I have followed if I had not been in a conventional and happy heterosexual relationship? I would certainly have at least sought the friendship of a young and dedicated runner, whether male or female. No anthropologist familiar with human history and the myriad human societies which peopled the world could think that love between two people of the same sex is abnormal or unnatural, whether expressed in emotional or physical terms. Love has too wide a meaning for such restrictive views, and religion must bear some of the blame for the hostility towards some natural forms of love.

I expected on my return to Ireland from my sojourn in Greece and France after I had left my family that I might not be welcomed by the hospital authorities, who were the Irish Sisters of Charity. I should have known better. As soon as I returned to Dublin, I had a call from the secretary manager, Sister Francis Joseph, welcoming me and insisting that I should attend a reception that was being held for some hospital event the following day. Many years later, when Louise, then a long-standing and greatly regarded ward sister in the hospital, and I married in a registry office, the sisters held a quiet reception for us in the convent. At one stage the head of the community took me aside and whispered in my ear, '*Isn't nice that we are getting a bit more sensible.*' I think the good nuns were willing to bend the rules as part of their concern for sinners as well as their appreciation of Louise's great contribution to the nursing services of the hospital.

My first contact with Louise Hederman was in July 1977 when, after a chance encounter in the hospital corridor, I invited her to play tennis in my club: she was chairperson of our hospital tennis club. It was the beginning of a warm relationship which was to blossom and to end in marriage in 1997 after twenty years of courtship. We married a few days after the divorce referendum had been passed. We had anticipated the result of the referendum in 1995, when we bought our home and went to live together. My invitation to tennis proved to have brought great happiness not only to me but to all my family. It was fortuitous but also cheeky as she was a much better player than me. She is now firmly established as the fount of knowledge and advice for family and friends on all medical and personal matters.

I think that my decision to leave my wife and to seek a divorce some years later also proved to be fortuitous. My children were generous in understanding my departure although at the time they had no idea of my motives in deserting the family.

My eldest boy, Richard, was the first to re-establish regular contact, but soon the rest came to visit me in my home in Lansdowne Lane, where they were generous in their acceptance of Jacqueline. I continued to visit Lissenfield every Saturday to care for the large garden and grounds. I was eventually invited in to the house with my usual basket of fruit for the children. A video, *Dan Dan, Dad and Me*, was created for RTÉ by my daughter and film director, Lisa, in later years; it portrayed the family fortunes, warts and all. It recalled my departure from the home, and included a film strip by Richard of the family's holiday activities in Connemara. Aileen had taken the entire family and some of their friends to a holiday beach there for the month following my departure. I was moved by the fact that, despite the loss and humiliation she must have suffered, she appeared to be fully involved in the festive activities. After her strenuous effort to save our marriage, she bore her loss with extraordinary equanimity and without a word of bitterness.

There was a gradual reconciliation over the ensuing years, finishing in the happy event of having Louise, with her nursing skills, looking after Aileen following a hip operation. Louise stayed with her in Aileen's home for ten days during early convalescence and was closely involved with Aileen during subsequent illnesses.

Aileen died in July 2008 after a long illness. She returned to her beloved Wexford, where she is buried near Bannow Bay, where the Normans landed in 1169. Thus ended our family saga: there was a full and happy reconciliation based on forgiveness by Aileen and our children. We learned a lot as a family. The lesson I learned was that a marriage which is not born in heaven may be best dissolved but that success in such a step depends on generosity and forgiveness on the part of parents and children, and understanding on the part of friends.

2

UNIVERSITY AND HOSPITAL TRAINING

I had left school just as the Second World War commenced. The majority of the Irish population was quite detached from the war; we might as well have been on another planet. We were most conscious of it during the Battle of Britain, the relatively short period of six to eight weeks in the summer of 1940 when there was extensive bombing of London and other British cities, including Belfast, and especially when we had one tragic bombing in Dublin. Every night we waited with excitement and apprehension for the first of the radio bulletins from London. For us it was by far the most dramatic and heroic episode of the war, at least until Stalingrad and the later period on the Eastern front.

My family and friends hoped that the Allies would win. Our hopes were strengthened when the Americans entered the war and when the Russian front opened in 1941. The rigours of shortages, the blackout and other restrictions increased as the war continued but I cannot say that we were any happier before or since. What we lacked in affluence and acquisitions we more than made up for in personal and collective security. There was no great public anxiety about invasion and no great dissatisfaction with living frugally and at times by our wits. Our local bicycle shop performed miracles in providing us with ersatz parts and repairs. Despite the six long years of war, the natural accumulation of articles and left-offs in attics, rubbish heaps, outhouses and garages provided some much-needed replacements for bicycle, sporting and household needs. One wonders how vast might be the accumulated items which could be utilised today in the event of the cutting-off of all supplies.

Transport was largely confined to the bicycle. The tramways provided a reasonable public transport system in Dublin but the countrywide rail system gradually deteriorated during the war and immediately afterwards because of the dearth of coal. Summer holidays consisted of cycling to Wexford, west Cork, Kerry and the west with a tent and our own cooking equipment. Bicycles were old and subject to many problems including broken chains, punctures and more serious damage or loss. Despite our impecunious state, the vagaries of the weather and some hardship, we seemed to enjoy these adventures. On one occasion we cycled the 130 miles from Galway to Dublin in eleven and a half hours with nothing worse than excoriated bottoms. On another, the crossbar of my ancient Raleigh broke and left me stranded in east Cork. I managed to get a lift on a turf lorry to Cork city, where I borrowed the money to take the train to Dublin. This was in 1944, when the railways had run out of coal and depended on turf. The locomotive needed to stop every twenty-five miles to clean out the massive amounts of residue of the peat from the furnace and to relight the fire and reheat the boiler. It took exactly twenty-four hours for the train to reach Dublin from Cork, a distance of 166 miles. Added to Scouting and rowing, such hardships must have made some contribution to my character, to my sense of independence and confidence.

Luxuries, including tobacco, alcohol and most imported products, were in increasingly short supply during and after the Emergency, as it was known in Ireland. At least there was no serious shortage of food. Indeed, the community benefited by a rationing system which ensured better nutrition for the poor. Before the war the Dublin artisan and working man and the unemployed were much smaller in stature compared to those of the middle classes, but this disparity began to diminish during wartime thanks to a more equal distribution of food. During the war, we were fortunate in Lissenfield to have our own fruit, vegetables and dairy foods.

THE UNIVERSITY

I was just turned seventeen when I entered medical school in September 1939. There were about 140 members in my class in University College Dublin. We were a motley crowd of callow youths, an unsophisticated lot, with about twenty women, who seemed shy and remote from the rest of us. At that time there were no restrictions in joining the medical faculty as long as one had passed the Leaving Certificate or the university entrance examination. However, a pass in Latin in the entrance examination was obligatory. This may seem an academic quirk to us nowadays, but perhaps the many medical words of Latin and Greek origin justified such a requirement. There was also a view in 1939, still lingering from earlier times, that a doctor should have a rounded education, which at that time would have included a familiarity with the classics. Unlike today's circumstances, when demand far exceeds places in medicine in all our universities, any person with a vocation for medicine and the necessary basic qualifications could enter the medical faculty.

The Earlsfort Terrace building always seemed crowded, particularly between lectures, and the institution lacked the traditional ambience of a university campus. It was often described at the time as a glorified technical college. The close-by Iveagh Gardens was our only open space and was available to the students and faculty, but in my time it was little used except as a means of walking the shortcut from the Earlsfort Terrace building to 85 and 86 St Stephen's Green. The latter buildings were the site of Newman's short-lived Catholic University, established in 1855 and still part of the university. (though it was moved in the 1960s from Earlsfort Terrace to the 'leafy suburbs' of south Dublin in Belfield). There we had the unlovely *aula maxima*, where we held our weekly 'hops', and the very lovely Newman Chapel.

My first three years were spent on this rather arid university campus, during which time we studied chemistry, physics, botany and zoology, and later anatomy, physiology and biochemistry. We had occasional lectures in medical ethics and jurisprudence. Towards the end of the third year, we attended a few clinical sessions in the hospitals. These first three years seem now, at least partly, a waste of time; the course could have been completed in half the time. Teaching was poor, at least in terms of stimulating our interest in these subjects, not because of their nature but because of the uninspired teaching which prevailed and the lack of intimate contact between faculty and students. My lack of interest was apparent from my poor examination results: I got a bare pass in each of the three examinations held during the three years.

I was fortunate to have had the distraction of the Boat Club during this time. It, and my delayed maturity, were probably responsible for my failure to face the academic challenge presented by third-level education. The uninspiring nature of my secondary education, with its failure to stimulate the natural creativity of young people, and its teaching by rote, contributed to my inability to take advantage of the university and to avail of its academic opportunities. The three years on the university campus could only retard and inhibit the naturally fertile mind of a young person.

I believe that after one academic year devoted to the basic scientific subjects (physics, chemistry and biology), medical students should continue their education, including applied physiology and anatomy, in the hospital and in the community. Beside the teaching of medicine by a skilled clinician, this could produce competent young doctors in substantially less time than the current five or six years of the curriculum. The thing that makes such a curriculum difficult is the unwillingness of general practitioners and consultants to devote the necessary time to teaching communication skills, patient management and clinical practice. We needed less pure science and more science applied to bedside practice.

During my campus years I had a knack for doing just enough work to scrape through my exams. The examination in June of the third year was the most important of these and was based on the complete anatomy, physiology and biochemistry courses. It was a busy year too in the rowing club. I realised coming close to the exam that I had done too little to hope to pass. I persuaded my reluctant parents to allow me to postpone the exam to September so that I could at the same time sit for the Henry Hutchinson medal and scholarship, which would eventually lead to the Fellowship of the Royal College of Surgeons, and no doubt to a brilliant career in surgery! My poor gullible parents were persuaded by the prospect of this galaxy of academic achievements. I breathed a sigh of relief, did the minimum amount of work during the summer after the rowing season was over, scraped through the exam in September, and promptly forgot about Henry Hutchinson and that brilliant career in surgery.

It was eight years later, in 1950, that I was to join the medical faculty of the same university, and thirty years later when I was to become professor of preventive cardiology. In later years too I became closely associated with the university historical archives as a trustee of the Mulcahy papers donated by my father to the university.

The first stirrings of my interest in medicine and in my future emerged in my fourth year in college, when we changed from the university campus to the hospital setting. This change in location and in the curriculum transformed my interest in medicine as a career. From this period onwards, I was satisfied that the profession which I had only casually chosen was the one that suited me best. Contact with doctors, nurses and patients had in immediate impact in giving me a feeling of belonging and participation. This was particularly emphasised when, later that year, we commenced our six-month residence as clinical clerks, part of the apprentice system of teaching which then prevailed in medicine in Dublin. We lived in the hospital student residence, becoming part of an active medical or surgical team. Although our duties were far from onerous, we did have an important role in taking histories from the patients and doing physical examinations, and also in providing a link between the patient and the visiting consultant. Our final three years were largely spent in the hospitals, where we commenced our clinical and bedside education. I managed an undistinguished second-class honours in my further examinations, moving from twelfth in the class in the third medical to eighth in the fourth and joint-second in the fifth and final examination. At no time did I show any academic brilliance, nor did I neglect my Boat Club commitments until my final year, when at last I put my oar away. The examinations mattered little as evidence of one's suitability for the practice of medicine, although at that time a brilliant examinee was virtually assured an appointment to one's teaching hospital as a consultant, subject to satisfying certain personality and social criteria in the perception of the hospital staff and owners.

St Vincent's Hospital

St Vincent's Hospital, which was to be my alma mater, was located at St Stephen's Green in a number of contiguous eighteenth-century Georgian buildings between Loreto College and Lower Lesson Street. It was of modest size with about 140 beds. It was unsuitable for a modern teaching hospital but it served its purpose at a time when there was little else to cater for except simple bedside and outpatient practice and relatively simple surgical procedures. Pathology and radiology were still a limited part of medical practice.

The hospital was established in 1832 by Mother Mary Aikenhead and the order she founded, the Sisters of Charity, to provide for the sick poor of the city. Support from the State for the public hospitals did not commence until after the war, so that they largely depended on private donations or on the income derived from the sweepstakes and private patients in the attached private nursing homes. St Vincent's was an intimate and friendly institution, as could be said for most of the small voluntary hospitals in Dublin at that time. It was administered by the Sisters, and in my student years had a relatively small consultant medical staff.

On my return there when I was appointed to the consultant staff in September 1950 there were six physicians. With the exception of the dermatologist and to a lesser extent the neurologist, all were general physicians and there was little evidence of the increasing trend to specialise in particular areas of internal medicine. One physician was appointed as professor to University College Dublin, close to St Vincent's at Earlsfort Terrace. There were five general surgeons, one of whom held a professorship at the university. We also had two radiologists, a dentist, a pathologist and a forensic pathologist, as well as an ear, nose and throat surgeon and an eye specialist. Previously anaesthetics were administered by the resident staff in the hospital and by general practitioners in the private surgical theatre. A trained anaesthetist was first appointed shortly after my departure from the resident staff in 1946. There was no psychiatrist; such problems were dealt with by the physician specialising in neurology, a common conjunction of practice at the time.

Teaching of undergraduates was based on the apprentice system. It was conducted at the bedside, with surgical classes, or 'clinics' as they were called, commencing at nine o'clock on the weekday mornings, and medical classes at ten. Attendances were not compulsory, so that the popularity of the teacher could be judged by the attendances at each class. It was a time in Dublin when the association between hospital and university was not as tight as it is today. It was then the tradition that students could wander as they pleased around the Dublin hospitals for the morning teaching clinics. A few of the UCD students were on the rolls of the Richmond, Jervis Street, Meath, Mercer's and Dr Steevens hospitals; but St Vincent's and Mater students could attend these and also Sir Patrick Dun's and Baggot Street for the morning teaching clinics. I seldom went outside St Vincent's except to attend teaching in the Richmond Hospital, where a renowned neurologist, Dr Harry Lee Parker, inspired in me a great interest in diseases of the nervous system. I rarely visited our sister hospital, the Mater, on the north side of the city.

Apart from my regular attendances at St Vincent's for clinical teaching, we were later obliged to visit other hospitals and institutions to qualify for certificates of competence in various disciplines which would permit us to sit the final examinations. I opted to go to Temple Street Children's Hospital to study paediatrics, to Grangegorman to hear John Dunne's lectures on the mental diseases, to Cork Street to learn about fevers, and to ear, nose and throat, and eye clinics. From each teacher we obtained certificates of competence, whether we had attended or not. In Grangegorman, which was the big municipal psychiatric hospital, we greatly enjoyed John Dunne's flamboyant presentations of his more bizarre patients. Dunne was an entertaining teacher (and eccentric member of my golf club) and I expect he was prone to exaggeration at times – as when he stated that a patient we saw with catatonic schizophrenia was transfixed and had not moved out of his chair for twenty years! Indeed, apart from attending Grangegorman, more out of morbid curiosity than any other reason, I don't think I attended more than a few of the other special lectures. I expect my rowing activities during term made such visits inconvenient, and, for the more impecunious students, the only mode of transport available was the bicycle. Each certificate cost three guineas, so that our teachers were not disadvantaged by our failure to attend their teaching sessions, and I expect that full attendances by a class of 140 students would anyway have been very inconvenient for them.

As a student I may have thought the standard of medical teaching was good in Dublin but in retrospect I was to change my views, on my arrival in London, when I found I had little insight into medical diagnosis and clinical methodology. The greatest shortcomings in the Dublin hospital scene, at least in the teaching of medicine as opposed to surgery, was that the teaching we received was rarely put into practice by the physicians who taught us. Precept yes, but example no. Lip service was paid to history-taking and comprehensive physical examination, but the physicians who taught me at St Vincent's had little training in clinical medicine, and most were appointed to the staff shortly after qualifying, without any extensive training abroad. On returning to Dublin in the autumn of 1950 fully trained in advanced clinical diagnosis of heart disease, I found that there was little knowledge of cardiac diagnosis and of the mechanism and significance of the signs elicited by the stethoscope, nor were my predecessors familiar with the precise clinical changes which occurred in patients with heart failure and heart irregularities.

The teaching of obstetrics, however, was a different matter as regards the seeking of special certificates before the final examination. Here, in order to earn one's certificate, it was necessary to attend and participate in twenty deliveries. To achieve this, it was mandatory to spend about two weeks in residence in the maternity hospital of one's choice. I attended the Coombe Lying-in Hospital. I went there with others from my class, including three Boat Club colleagues – to ensure that our social activities were not neglected. We occupied cubicles in a residence which was sparse and primitive in the extreme, but this caused us no hardship as they were well up to the standards we were accustomed to at that time.

The first two of our twenty assigned deliveries took place in the labour ward, where the nursing staff and residents instructed us in the delivery of a baby. Here we were expected to learn all the mysteries of confinement and childbirth, and the immediate hazards to which the mother and child are exposed. Nor was the spiritual side neglected: we were informed that, should the baby be dead on delivery, or expire shortly afterwards, a simple ritual of baptism was obligatory if the newborn was not to spend the rest of eternity in that godforsaken place, Limbo.

Having witnessed the first two deliveries, we were now on our own. Students were paired and the next eighteen deliveries were carried out on the district, that is, in the homes of the expectant mothers. The Coombe was close to the Liberties and right in the middle of some of Dublin's worst slums. Many of these home deliveries took place there. All were conducted by the students but in the event of difficulties we were obliged to call for assistance by the junior resident doctor, or clinical clerk, on call. He would then deal with the problem in the patient's house and if necessary he would have her transferred to the hospital to be managed by the assistant master or the master himself.

It must seem incredible that students could be thrown in at the deep end in that way when the lives of both mother and child were at stake. But there were some fail-safe factors to protect the mother and child. There was invariably a midwife or experienced handywoman present from the neighbourhood to deal with routine deliveries. The fact that childbirth was a natural process was a further protection, provided we did not interfere with the natural course of affairs. Finally, there was always recourse to the medical staff in the hospital in case of complications or emergencies. The system of student attendance at home births would not be tolerated nowadays, and anyway the ubiquitous spread of medical litigation in recent years would preclude such an arrangement, but in the 1940s, 1930s and earlier, the system served the communities of the city well.

The circumstances of the poor in the slums were appalling. To those of us coming from middle-class homes, the impact of their conditions on us was quite traumatic. I recall an early visit to a slum dwelling near the hospital in Thomas Street. It was an old dilapidated Georgian house of three storeys over basement. There was no front door. The timberwork of the hallway and stairs was rotten, with missing planks and holes in abundance. We had to climb to the second floor with the greatest care to avoid falling into the basement. Part of the banisters was missing and there was no sign of a stick of proper furniture in the patient's wretched two rooms. However, the worst feature was the appalling smell: the bitter, acrid, penetrating smell which we learnt emanated from crushed bed bugs, which were a ubiquitous feature of the Dublin slums.

The patient was multiparous – that is, she had had numerous pregnancies and many children. She was obese, malodorous and filthy, and must have rarely washed herself. She lay naked on sackcloth on an old trestle bed, crying out with pain and scarcely aware of what was happening around her. It was an incredible picture of poverty, filth and neglect; and all about her, in the two rooms they occupied, were her unkempt children and her husband. His only contribution to the affair was to express his admiration for us two boys that we could resist the alluring prospect and joys of her nether region, confessing that he had always found her irresistible! And all the time it took me every effort not to vomit.

This description may seem exaggerated to those who never entered the old Dublin slums, but every student who went through the Coombe will testify to such experiences. The filth, degradation and poverty are fortunately things of the past in Ireland; it is not necessary to be reminded of the improvement of the conditions of the underprivileged in the city and in the country. It is at the same time salutary to remember that these people, despite their material degradation, were part of a tightly knit community and enjoyed some compensations, such as their faith and their own code of behaviour. Indeed, when they were provided with new homes after the war, in what were then outer suburbs, many were reluctant to go and were only compelled to do so because of the dereliction or demolition of the tenements.

We had many odd moments and experiences in the Coombe while out on the district. On one occasion when called, my partner and I were told to attend a confinement in a house above Haffner's shop in South Great George's Street. Haffner's was famous for its sausages and will be remembered for the perpetual queue outside its door. We entered the first floor and went directly into the patient's room from a fire escape at the back of the building. The patient appeared to be alone in the house; she was sitting up in the bed, dressed in black a negligee, and very composed considering that she was in labour. There was a curious stillness about the place, but soon we were joined by the midwife, who entered from another room. She led us back into this adjoining room where we found the patient's husband – dead and laid out in a coffin. It was a rather bizarre and macabre sight, and there was a strangeness about the patient's perfect state of composure, despite the two crises which she was facing. Perhaps she felt that she was merely swapping one person for another!

It was at the end of November that I and my partner made our first domiciliary visit. It was late on a Saturday or, rather, early on Sunday morning. It was 1944 and the blackout in the city was complete. We were called to a house in Crumlin. We were unfamiliar with the topography of the area and we had the greatest difficulty in finding the correct address. We must have been cycling around the suburb for two hours or more before we eventually got to our patient. The midwife was there encouraging the lady to bear down, that is, to strain and to do everything she could to extrude the infant. The pain continued for the rest of the night and into the morning, without any visible results. We thought it wise to stay by her and miss Sunday mass in case she should deliver the child, and we waited patiently until late on Sunday evening.

The episodic pain continued but there was no sign of the baby. Eventually, early on Monday morning, in desperation I returned to the hospital to report to the clinical clerk, a particularly difficult and irascible character who was not more than two years qualified. He refused to visit the woman but suggested that we should administer an enema. I was provided with the necessary equipment and given brief advice about its use. Back I went and we administered the enema, but in doing so we made a frightful mess of the poor woman's bed and room. Clearly the liquid had not been administered in the correct manner, and later, during a particularly abrasive altercation with the clinical clerk, we were accused of having administered the enema into the wrong orifice, a possibility which had already occurred to us.

The woman's pains persisted until early on Tuesday morning, when they gradually subsided. We returned to the hospital to be abused and savaged by the clinical clerk again, who demanded to know if we had ever heard of constipation. In retrospect I feel that he was a little hard on us as this was the first confinement which we had conducted – or at least hoped to conduct. She was eventually delivered about ten days later by two other students who were in residence with us.

We had been more than forty-eight hours attending our first domiciliary call and got no credit for our trouble. The clinical clerk had a most lurid and colourful vocabulary which he employed freely when addressing the nurses, patients and students. He was testy in the extreme and he had the shortest fuse of anybody I have ever known. Despite these rather unusual professional traits, he was an excellent doctor and was subsequently well known and greatly respected as a general practitioner in the Midlands. Because of our long first case, and perhaps too because of some prolonged sessions in the local pub, I had only delivered thirteen patients during the allotted two weeks. In order to complete my full complement of twenty deliveries and thus qualify to do my final examination, I returned to the Coombe at Christmas, when fewer students were likely to be there. I delivered the remaining seven women in three days. Happily our twenty deliveries were achieved without mishap, a tribute no doubt to the midwives and to the fundamental role of nature, but hardly to our own very limited interventions.

While in residence we were expected to attend the master's lectures and ward rounds each day. However, most of my time was spent on the district and not infrequently in the local pub, known by generations of Coombe students as the 'PPH', named after 'postpartum haemorrhage', or for the initiated, the 'pub past hospital'. About seven or eight days after my arrival in the Coombe, I left the residency to cross the yard to Number 8, one of the labour wards. I saw this rather tubby, immaculately groomed gentleman attempting to swing the starting handle of a Rolls Royce in the yard. I offered to lend a hand and after a few attempts by me the great machine purred into action. The owner thanked me warmly and kindly asked me my name and my purpose in visiting the hospital. I explained that I was a resident student completing my obstetrical education. It transpired, of course, that he was the master and that not only had I failed to attend his teaching sessions, but I had not even met him before this occasion. He was kindness itself in gently admonishing me and expressed the hope that we would meet again before my obstetrical education was completed. He was Dr Ned Keelan, the gentlest and kindest of men, and a striking contrast to the aforementioned clinical clerk. I expect the master was terrified of his junior colleague!

In 1944 the shortages caused by the war were impinging more on our lives. The shortages included those of many alcoholic drinks. In the PPH the only drink available was Guinness or Portuguese brandy. The draught Guinness, or 'pint of plain' at that time, varied greatly in quality, depending on a number of factors, including the expertise of the publican, the cleanliness of the process and the equipment employed to store and dispense it. The bottle of stout was much more popular at that time because of the wide variation in the quality of the draught brew.

My usual drink was fifty-fifty, a bottle of stout added to a half-pint of plain. At times, when the Guinness was exhausted, we were obliged to drink the Portuguese brandy. This particular fire-water had obviously been in the pub long before the war started. The bottle was old and dust-covered, and was fetched from the highest shelf. The constraints of wartime must have been a heaven-sent opportunity for the publican to jettison his ancient stock; nor were we particularly reluctant to help him do so.

In the pub we met some of the local men, most of whom had had their children delivered by the students from the Coombe. We were always addressed as 'doctor', a title which was a considerable source of gratification to us. In fact, the Coombe and its cohort of student *accoucheurs* were highly regarded by the local community. At that time, if anything went wrong during a delivery it was viewed philosophically as a misfortune, as an act of God and an expression of His will, and not as an opportunity to seek financial compensation. At the time the annual indemnity insurance was not more than £2; today the obstetricians pay £200,000 or more.

Behind the earthiness and informality of the Coombe façade which I have described, and despite the participation of scantily trained students in the day-to-day work of the hospital, Dublin and Irish obstetrics have a history and tradition which must always be a source of pride and international recognition to Ireland. I was pleased to be appointed to the Coombe as a physician and cardiologist in 1950 when I returned to Dublin from London, and I continued in that position until I retired from hospital practice in October 1988. I enjoyed the clinical work there and it provided opportunities for research into the influence of smoking by mothers on the health of the baby. It also provided an opportunity to research the treatment of high blood pressure in mothers, a condition which can lead to serious consequences for both mother and child. I was joined with my previous resident, John Murphy, and a few others in these projects, which would later lead to nine publications in the Irish, British and American medical press.

The strength of Dublin obstetrics and our maternity hospitals was based on the mastership system. The Rotunda was founded by Bartholomew Mosse in 1735 and the Coombe and National Maternity Hospitals were founded in the nineteenth century. All three hospitals were controlled by a master, who was always an experienced obstetrician and who had considerable power over his colleagues. He played a major role in managing the hospital and formulating policy. The appointment lasted seven years and could not be renewed. On only one occasion in the cumulative five hundred years of the three hospitals was the seven-year rule broken: John Cunningham, master of the National Maternity Hospital in the 1940s, required an Act of Parliament to allow him two additional years to complete the commissioning of the new hospital in Holles Street.

The master was a virtual dictator during his seven years but he returned to the ranks afterwards. I believe the advantages accruing from effective and unimpeded decision-making, which was implicit in the system, far outweighed the possible disadvantages accruing from the rare appointment of an unsuitable candidate. I also believe that all members of the medical profession should be subjected to peer review; this is an integral feature of the mastership system. The international recognition of Dublin as a maternity centre of excellence was partly based on the mastership tradition and also based on the tradition of audit (whereby it was mandatory for the master to produce an annual report containing all details of his stewardship and appropriate statistics, including detailed infant and maternal morbidity and mortality data). These reports were presented each year for professional and public discussion at a specially convened meeting of the Royal Irish Academy of Medicine, where the three masters presented their reports and where criticism was often frank, outspoken and constructive.

The mastership system also ensured that professional problems, including potentially damaging interpersonal conflicts between members of the hospital staff, were solved within the profession. Today, when we recall a few debacles in our general hospitals involving such conflicts and possible recourse to the law courts, the mastership system of limited tenure and professional responsibility in some form is urgently needed. A chief of staff with responsibility, executive power, and limited tenure, elected by his peers and with time to devote to administration as well as professional practice, is needed if the medical profession is to continue to order its own affairs, to play its vital role in hospital administration, and to protect its reputation among the public.

UNIVERSITY DAYS

During my first year in university I weighed six stone and measured five feet two inches in height. Because of my diminutive size and my child-like appearance, I was reasonably popular in my class, mainly because of my peers' curiosity at my physical retardation. I was treated to some extent as a mascot, as if I were attached to a football team. A family friend, a boxing enthusiast and general practitioner in Enniscorthy, Bob Bowe, tried hard to induce me to join the boxing club on my arrival in the university as a flyweight; but competition from the Boat Club, always seeking pygmy specimens as a cox, won the day. My diminutive physique was the source of almost paternalistic affection on the part of my hefty rowing companions during my first year or two in the Boat Club.

I cannot recall whether I was anxious about my belated physical development when I first went to college but I was certainly immature in terms of confidence and personality. My lack of confidence may have been partly due to my physique but I was also affected by my being pitched from the ambience of an Irish-speaking secondary school, with its post-Civil War illiberal political and cultural background, including its strict prohibition of 'foreign games', into the middle of that wider spectrum of people from the larger English-speaking schools, with their perceived sophistication and wider and more liberal sporting and cultural backgrounds. I was far too conscious of my Irish-Ireland background to speak at any of the college society meetings, such as the Literary and Historical Society or the Medical Society, which were such an important element of our university experience. This may account for a certain diffidence and lack of confidence in future years in speaking off the cuff to an audience. I was certainly intimidated by some aspects of my early college life but my confidence grew as I made a niche for myself in the Boat Club and as I established friendships with members of my class and with many outside my own faculty. I was greatly helped to overcome my inferiority complex by my putting on nine or ten inches in height during my second year. My sudden sprouting was as much a surprise to myself as it was to others, and, although I soon exceeded the ideal weight of a cox, I was still skeleton-thin and I continued as cox of the senior eight for a third year. It was only in my fourth year in college that I was deemed robust enough to be an oarsman.

During my third year I was appointed secretary of the Students' Representative Council, my first essay into politics and no doubt evidence of some political genes. As representatives of the students, my colleagues and I acted as a link between the students and the university authorities. However, my main function was to allot the Friday night dances, or 'hops', to the different student societies. This gave me considerable influence because the societies needed the receipts from the hops to pay their very modest expenses. I took advantage of my position to gain free admission to the dances and, although I did not drink at the time, I accepted whatever other hospitality was available on these occasions. It was the first occasion in which I was exposed to the temptations of power and corruption.

I recall the circumstances under which we lived, and indeed thrived, when I was a member of the Boat Club. While preparing for each regatta, we would go into training for periods of up to six weeks – no smoking or alcohol, no association with the opposite sex (although this was for all of us surely an academic restriction) and bed before eleven o'clock. There was a strict code of honour which obliged us to obey these orders. We usually trained six days every week. For me it was a three-mile cycle up the Grand Canal to the clubhouse in Islandbridge, often into the prevailing wind, and sometimes in hail, rain or snow. We changed in a draughty and unheated pavilion, and rowed two or three times up and down the Liffey between Chapelizod and the weir at Islandbridge, a distance of just over one mile. Afterwards we threw ourselves into cold showers before cycling the three miles back to Rathmines. Rarely would I take the Lucan tram which clattered along the road by the clubhouse, as this was a luxury I could not often afford. It was one of the larger double-decker trams, equipped with a double set of bogies, and designed for the longer distances to the outer suburbs at Lucan, Dalkey and Howth. I recall the powerful clattering rhythm of this great beast as it left the city precincts at Islandbridge and set off for the long haul to our clubhouse and beyond to Lucan. While by the modern standards of the motor car it hardly travelled very fast, it gave an impression of speed and power because of its bulk and the clattering noise of the bogies.

To the present-day student, ours may have seemed a spartan way of life with a masochistic love of physical hardship, but at the time we had no great feelings of suffering. Physical exercise was a routine part of our lives then, and to all of us the bicycle and the tram were the only means of transport. I don't think I ever missed a training session, whether as a cox or oarsman, at least without giving adequate notice of my absence. To fail to turn up would leave the other members of the crew in the lurch. Of all sports, rowing is the one where the individual is totally subordinated by the group. It was a wonderful training, not only in achieving physical fitness but also in inculcating a spirit of camaraderie and loyalty to the group. My experience in the Boat Club, and my earlier experience in the Boy Scouts, played a major part in the development of my character, and in preparing me for a career in medicine. In those earlier years, I learnt the satisfaction to be derived from working and serving with others.

Once or twice we missed practice because the river was frozen. On one such occasion five of us took our bikes out on the iced river and cycled the short mile up to Chapelizod and back. There is no doubt that such adventures are part of the intrepid lives of the young, and in retrospect it makes me wonder how I could take such risks. The icing of rivers and lakes was not unusual at that time but is no longer seen in our recent mild winters and springs, a reminder no doubt of the advance of climate change.

The Boat Club was housed in a low, single-storey clubhouse on the north bank of the River Liffey just beyond Islandbridge. It was built in the early thirties and was replaced about twenty-five years ago by a much more palatial building on a different site. The old pavilion consisted of a large room with locker seats along the walls. There was a toilet and two showers at one end. It was a draughty building with concrete block walls and the steel windows which were a feature of many buildings, including private houses, before the war. These windows invariably seemed to buckle with time, and the Boat Club pavilion was no exception to this. I have memories of lockers with ancient togs, some of which had long since been abandoned by their owners. While apparently abandoned, they did occasionally come in handy for those of us who had forgotten our shorts, singlets or socks, or who had on those rare occasions left them to be laundered or repaired. It appears that our rugged way of life at that time protected us from being too squeamish.

During practice sessions, we appeared in an extraordinary variety of rowing togs. Being before the age of disposables, and because of the rigours and shortages of war, new togs were an unaccustomed luxury. However at regatta times we appeared pristine and neat in our singlets with the UCD crest over the left breast, and with shorts and socks to match. We would emulate our Trinity College peers on such occasions, with their long tradition of sartorial elegance; we in our dark blue blazers (for maidens and juniors) or light blue (for seniors who had been awarded the university colours) and flannel trousers and scarf. The longer and more voluminous the scarf, the greater the ease of having it hanging from the neck in front and back, and the closer we came to the sartorial elegance of the Trinity oarsmen.

On the wall facing the entrance to the locker room of our pavilion was a fine bronze plaque commemorating the name and munificence of Professor Arthur Clery, who had been a KC in the British time, but who had never practised in the Irish courts after the Treaty. He was a bachelor and obviously wealthier than most academics attached to the university. He had died some years before I reached college in 1939, but Clery had apparently made it possible to build the Club pavilion through his generous gift to the college and the Boat Club. He approved of rowing as a sport for young men but he apparently espoused certain standards of behaviour among the rowing fraternity. One condition attached to his gift prohibited the consumption of alcoholic beverages on the premises. This unfortunate restriction presented the members of the club, and indeed our many graduates and alickadoos who came to support us at regatta time, with a serious dilemma. Most nights after a regatta in Dublin, we would finish our celebrations in Islandbridge after we had been ejected from the bona fide public house at the closing hour of midnight. We had no other place to retire to from the pub; and whether we had sojourned in Matt Smith's or the Widow Flavin's in Sandyford, the Dead Man's in Palmerston or the Fisherman's Rest in Castleknock, we would return to the clubhouse to continue our celebrations, where we might still be found long after dawn singing the traditional scatological songs and limericks of the rowing world. The problem of Arthur Clery's prohibition on alcohol was solved by the ritual of hanging a towel over the plaque, which remained *in situ* until the last bottle of Guinness had been consumed.

We were no different, then, from many other undergraduates who appeared to relax by letting their hair down at the end of the day of competition. I had never tasted an alcoholic drink until I had completed my third year in college, but this did not in any way affect my participation in these nocturnal celebrations. Guinness was almost exclusively the drink; the pint of draught in the pubs and bottled Guinness in the clubhouse. Some had incredible capacities for this drink, and post-regatta competitions of various sorts were the rule, either to test one's total capacity or to find the macho type who could drink a pint the fastest. Timing was from the moment the glass was lifted to the moment it was replaced on the table, emptied of all its contents. Dribbling disqualified, as did repeated retching or regurgitation. I think the record was twelve seconds flat. This was recorded one night in Trinity and it was, I think, achieved by a slim Trinity type. He must have had on oesophagus the diameter of a three-inch pipe!

Amateur sport was truly amateur sixty years ago. Sponsorship was unknown. Apart from a modest annual grant from the university authorities, which went to pay for new equipment and repairs, all expenses related to entrance fees to regattas and travelling were paid by ourselves, or rather our parents. Every year, apart from the Wylie Cup, Head of the River, Trinity, and the Metropolitan regattas in Dublin, we would travel to at least one regatta in the provinces – Limerick and Cork generally and occasionally to Galway, Drogheda, Belfast (despite the war) and Killarney. For events outside Dublin, boats – two fours and two eights – were placed and secured on a railway flat car and generally were handled by ourselves.

Once every year during the August holiday weekend, and after the official rowing season was over for the universities, some of us would set off the one hundred miles on our old bikes late on Friday to participate in the last and most famous regatta of the season at Carrick-on-Shannon, where we would sleep rough. The distance travelled was important for impoverished oarsmen because it was a rule of the IARU, the rowing authority in Ireland, that the entrance fee was waived for those oarsmen who were obliged to travel one hundred miles or more. We would borrow a boat during the regatta and participate in one or two races, retire afterwards to a pub or appropriate hostelry for a long night of celebration and revelry, and mount our bikes two mornings later for our slow return to

Dublin. We sometimes had to return sooner because funds were generally so low after the night's celebrations that we couldn't afford to eat. At that time there were many lorries travelling between Dublin and the provinces carrying turf or peat – the only available fuel during the Emergency. We were fortunate on some occasions to meet such lorries and to have ourselves and our bikes accommodated on top of the load of turf. This was long before the anti-drink-driving campaigns were introduced and the lorry drivers were generally glad to accommodate us and to join us in the odd pub or shebeen on the way.

My alcohol-free life ended after a Boat Club regatta in Drogheda. It was a particularly stormy day, with heavy seas running at the mouth of the Boyne estuary, where each race started. The one-and-a-half-mile race finished close to the great Boyne railway viaduct. I was coxing the senior eight. The maiden-eight cox was a first-year student without much experience, and it was not surprising that he lost his nerve when he encountered the turbulent waters of the River Boyne. I was obliged to take out six boats in all, but in five races we failed to finish after becoming swamped by the huge swell. We were quite safe of course thanks to the buoyancy compartments of the boat, and the eight oars.

Nonetheless it was a nerve-racking and hypothermic experience, and by the end of the afternoon I was both physically and mentally affected by the prolonged exposure. It was at this stage that I was induced to take a glass of whiskey. Its immediate restorative effects encouraged me to have another, and as the euphoria increased my discretion diminished, so that within an hour, and long before the regatta dinner started, I became violently ill and had to be transported to my hotel bed, where I slept it off over the next twelve hours. Unfortunately, instead of swearing off alcohol forever, as one might expect after such an experience, I never looked back. Except for short and isolated periods, I never returned to my teetotaller days.

I recall how impecunious I was during my first few years in college. Pocket money was understandably meagre considering that my father's total income from his Dáil salary and military pension hardly reached £700 annually. My lack of money did not appear to have any adverse effect on my life, but I was fortunate in that I took little or no alcohol during my first three years, I did not smoke regularly and I had no girlfriend to lavish money on.

During my first year or two, the only source of regular income was my visits to the Theatre Royal matinée every Friday afternoon with three friends. The Theatre Royal was demolished about forty-five years ago to make way for Hawkins House, the inelegant headquarters of the Department of Health. It was by far the largest cinema in Dublin then and since, with seating for more than two thousand. It was unique in the city in providing a continuous two-feature programme including film and stage show.

The stage show was made famous by Noel Purcell, who provided comedy; by Eddie Byrne, who conducted Question Time; and by the Royalettes, twelve gorgeous creatures, gaudily but lightly clad and showing the maximum amount of flesh which contemporary cultural constraints and the Catholic Archbishop, John Charles McQuaid, would allow. There was also a full feature film, the Movietone News, and sometimes other short film features.

Byrne was probably the first entertainer to introduce Question Time, at least in Ireland. He would invite four members of the audience up to the stage. The prize was ten shillings and it was awarded to the person who answered the most questions correctly. In the case of a tie, the money was divided. We always went on the Friday afternoon because we had usually tired of lectures by the end of the week – or perhaps our teachers had not lasted the pace – and the price of admission was only one shilling for the matinées. We sat to the front of the parterre and as soon as Eddie appeared we would rush up to the stage and take our places. Occasionally somebody else from the audience would beat us to it, or our foursome might not all be present. However, thanks to our combined knowledge and our military efficiency, we never failed to win the prize, even when we were not at full strength. Joe McHale, one of my threesome, was well informed and had quick reactions. He was to become an international at tennis and bridge, and was the bulwark of our group.

The occasional stray who would beat us to the stage invariably invoked our contempt because of his ignorance. We could scarcely conceal our amusement when they would commit a howler, such as the answer to the question, 'What is the highest obelisk in the world?' The answer Eddie sought was the Wellington Monument in the Phoenix Park, but the igno-ramus, after much head-scratching and a little prompting from Eddie, answered 'Mount Everest'! I think Eddie must have forgotten the Washington Monument in Washington, D.C.! We each left the theatre, one and sixpence the richer and after a full afternoon's entertainment. This was enough for me to pay the odd tram fare and other minor expenses. We did attempt to go a second time in one week but we were discouraged by Eddie, who thought we were just being greedy.

The Royalettes danced, threw their legs in strict unison and generally cavorted about the stage without apparently stimulating any untoward or lascivious reactions among my friends and myself. I think that we were probably too concerned about our commercial undertaking to respond much to their allurements. It should not be thought that we had no contact with the Royalettes. They not infrequently invited members of the audience to join them in various dances and other frivolities. The first time I saw or even heard of the Boomps-a-Daisy was one Friday afternoon. After several demonstrations of the dance by the well-trained, enticing group, I was one of the volunteers who agreed to participate in a pro-am performance. While my memory of the event is far from clear, I found myself embracing this gorgeous creature. We did a twirl, bowed and finished each movement by striking our buttocks together, although, to be more exact, she did most of the striking. She was rather stocky and smaller than the other girls but what she lacked in stature she made up for in muscle and strength. She reminded me a little of a weightlifter. At the end of the dance, her buttock met mine with enough energy to send me flying and staggering around the stage. I was dazed by the assault and, being slow to leave the stage with the other participants, I was struck on the head by the heavy descending curtain, adding to my disorientation. Anxious stage-hands rushed to my aid, I was bundled backstage and, shortly afterwards and much to my embarrassment, I was pushed out into the auditorium through a side door, none the worse for wear, apart from a tender right ischial tuberosity ('bum' in popular parlance).

During my fourth year in college, my mother procured a part-time job for me with the *Sunday Independent*. These part-time jobs were very difficult to find at that time of limited employment and of need; and no doubt I was doing some employee of the newspaper out of a few extra bob to support wife and family. The editor was an admirer of my father's and was apparently badgered by my mother into employing me. I worked at the newspaper's office in Middle Abbey Street from six to ten o'clock every Monday evening opening the envelopes and checking the contents of the entries for the *Sunday Independent* crossword, which was then very popular, with its weekly prize of £500. For four hours on Wednesday night we would check the valid coupons seeking the winning solution. It was repetitive and boring work, and required careful attention to avoid missing a correct coupon, but it paid me valuable pocket money for about a year, and sustained me as one of the wealthiest in my class. I was paid ten shillings each night and, at busy times, I might do overtime and get extra money. From being one of the poorest in the class, I became one of the more affluent, a circumstance that ensured my popularity with my peers was greatly enhanced.

Dennis McCullough was my godfather and was married to Agnes Ryan, my mother's sister. He was an ardent Irish nationalist from the North who had founded the republican Dungannon Clubs there, and had been chairman of the secret separatist group, the Irish Republican Brotherhood, up to the time of the Rising. McCullough was a prudent but generous godfather. I don't think he ever forgot my birthday, at least up to my twenty-first. This birthday, however, proved to be a rather embarrassing occasion. He sent for me on 13 July 1943, and presented me with a £5 note, a considerable sum and a generous gift at that time. He complimented me on my record in the university, emphasising in particular that I a gave good example to his two boys by not smoking and drinking. His two boys, Mairtin and Donncha, were younger than me and had followed me into UCD and the Boat Club. In fact, I was drinking and smoking by this time, but I had concealed the fact from my parents and the older generation. Nor did I think it an opportune moment to confess these sins to my godfather. Naturally, I did not wish to upset him and, most of all, I did not wish to jeopardise the financial donation he had made to me.

I was greatly comforted by the sudden improvement in my finances, and, in this moment of gratitude and elation, I invited my two Boat Club friends, Des Hogan and Kapo O'Sullivan, to join me next morning in Davy Byrne's for a pint. Not being regatta time and not being in training, we were free to enjoy a smoke and a few drinks. We were comfortably ensconced with our cigarettes and pints in the snug at the back of Davy

Byrne's, with its discrete entrance from the adjoining lane, when the door opened and in came M. W. O'Reilly, the chief executive of the New Ireland Assurance, followed by the chairman of the board of directors, Dennis McCullough! My poor godfather was struck dumb. He stared unbelievably at me and my pint, stood transfixed for what seemed an interminable time, and, after a strangled and disapproving grunt, followed slowly after M.W. into the front lounge of the pub. We stayed where we were even if it was for me only a question of drowning my sorrows. I had a bizarre notion for a while that he might demand his money back.

At first I thought his state of shock and dismay was caused by the sudden revelation that, rather than being the paragon he thought, I appeared to be well on the road to ruin. However, later and on more mature reflection, I realised that his upset may have been caused by his having to take his morning drink in the main bar, where he would certainly be seen by his employees from the nearby New Ireland offices. He was a man who, at least in social matters, liked to keep a low profile. Although prudent in his habits, and concerned always about his reputation of middle-class respectability, he enjoyed his occasional glass of malt and was one of the few who was offered his favourite brew during visits to my home.

I am not too sure that my parents were aware of my newly acquired taste for alcoholic beverages. Shortly after the birthday in question I had been out with my Boat Club friends when we finished the night in the well-known bona fide house of Matt Smith in Sandyford. Here we were more than three miles from our homes and could, according the law of the time, be classified as travellers. We were thus allowed to drink in a pub until midnight, although the normal pubs were obliged to close at ten o'clock in the winter and ten-thirty in the summer. It was one of those quaint laws which were a feature of Ireland before we joined the European Union and began to conform to international customs.

I arrived back at about half-past twelve at the gates of Lissenfield where, before venturing up the long avenue, I carefully inspected the house for signs of life. Much to my surprise, I found the lights still on in the drawing room: my parents were obviously burning the midnight oil. I waited, but shortly afterwards the lights were extinguished and I had only to wait until the lights appeared in my parents' bedroom. I then went up the avenue, opened the door quietly with my key, and stepped into the hallway. Again, much to my surprise, I found my parents climbing the stairs – they had obviously returned downstairs for same purpose or another. As they turned towards the top of the stairs to greet me, my mother said 'Is that you, Risteárd?' and I decided, being a man of quick action and intelligence, that I would do something which I might normally do if I were sober. I thought of the grandfather clock on the other side of the hall: it surely needed winding. I walked briskly and without hesitation over to the clock, swung open the hinged window protecting the clock face, pulled it off its hinges and sent it flying across the hallway with a crash and the sound of splintering grass which, to my ears, would have wakened the dead.

My parents stood riveted at the top of the stairs for what seemed an interminable period of time. I must have been wide-mouthed and imbecilic, and equally riveted, below them. To their eternal credit, they broke the silence by saying 'Goodnight', and continued on their way to the next landing and to their bedroom. This, I can say, was the most embarrassing experience of my life.

During my final year as a student I stopped rowing and devoted most of my time to the hospital and to study. My final examination was complicated by the fact that I suffered from severe writer's cramp as a result of rowing in the number two stroke position on the UCD junior eight in 1944. In the early summer of 1944, I noticed rapid wasting of the thenar muscles in my right hand, the large muscle mass at the base of the thumb. I had developed what was later called the median nerve syndrome, where the nerve to the muscle is damaged in its passage under the fibrous sheath at the wrist. It was caused by the pressure exerted on the nerve as I feathered the heavy oar with my right hand. The condition slowly resolved over a few months after the rowing season came to an end, but I was left with a severe writer's cramp which had shown little improvement by the late spring of 1945, when I sat the final medical examination. To this day I cannot understand how the examiners could read my indecipherable script. They must have had some intuitive insight into my state of knowledge or must have considered that I was an eminently suitable person to write prescriptions in the real tradition of the profession! Somebody once aptly suggested that I write in Braille!

Later, in 1948, when I sat the London membership examination, I wrote reams of stuff at the two essay sessions, but during the last few moments of each session, when I had a quick look over what I had written, I was unable to read my own writing. My writing never recovered from the apparent temporary damage to the median nerve, although the cramp has largely resolved, except when my hand becomes fatigued after prolonged scribbling or when I use the hand for unusual heavy work. I probably succeeded in passing the membership examination of the London College of Physicians in 1948 because I used frequent titles or headings in capitals, thus conveying some inkling to the examiner of what was in my mind.

POSTGRADUATE AND HOSPITAL RESIDENCY

I qualified as a doctor in June 1945. At this important juncture in my life I informed my parents that I wished to remain independent of them financially. They therefore arranged for me to have a £500 overdraft facility. It was a measure of the bank's regard for my parents that the manager accepted their role as guarantors, although they had an unsecured overdraft in another bank which they only succeeded in clearing in the 1950s, when ministerial pensions were introduced. I suppose I should be grateful that I have lived long enough since then to have paid sixty-five premiums of five pounds. At least my beneficiaries will eventually receive the equivalent of five hundred Irish pounds.

I was appointed resident house surgeon to Frank 'Pops' Morrin at St Vincent's Hospital and later house physician to the professor of medicine, Donagh O'Donovan, newly returned from Canada. The physicians at St Vincent's were a conservative, conventional and sober group. The surgeons were a more flamboyant lot and their teaching was less academic and had a more practical basis. Harry Meade, the professor of surgery, was effective through his constant reiteration of the basic principles of surgical diagnosis, while Bill Doolin was arresting to us callow lot because of his florid language, his carefully manicured diction, his frequent literary allusions (by then going out of fashion), and his aquiline appearance evocative of a Roman emperor. Bob O'Connell had the necessary flamboyance to attract students, and Paddy FitzGerald, later to succeed Harry Meade as professor of surgery, was quiet and measured of speech and slow and meticulous of action, and was an excellent if somewhat arid teacher. Jamsie Maher, bachelor, chain smoker (and sadly to prove an early victim of the habit, like many of his colleagues) and football alickadoo, was always late and could often be found doing rounds in the nursing homes after midnight. He was a lovable, eccentric and popular figure but a dangerous host – he would often lock the door of his house in Fitzwilliam Place to prevent us from going home long after the bewitching hour. He first introduced me to the Guinness and champagne mix, appropriately called Black Velvet. I first saw the *Sputnik* in orbit in the early morning as I sojourned there and I was not a little embarrassed to meet my father at seven o'clock in the morning on our avenue on his way to mass nearby. He passed me by with a brisk 'Good morning'!

'Pops' Morrin was trained in the trenches during the Great War and joined the Irish army during the Civil War. He was one of three or four doctors in the army medical corps who afterwards joined the staffs of our teaching hospitals. My father spoke highly of their service to the rapidly expanding infant army and maintained that they had organised an excellent medical service under the most difficult circumstances. A man of few words, and sharp ones at that, Morrin was the master of emergency surgery but paid little attention to the academic side of his profession or even to patient after-care. I worked with him later as a physician. He was glad to pass all non-surgical procedures to me or other members of the staff.

A young man was admitted to the surgical ward in an exsanguinated condition (that is, he was losing blood) with a ruptured kidney after having been run over by a cart. Fortunately, Morrin and I were doing rounds and were immediately at hand. The semi-conscious patient was manhandled by Morrin, who, with some assistance, rushed him down to the nearby surgical theatre. He tore the patient's blood-soaked clothes off him as he shouted at me to start the anaesthetic. I clapped the Clover apparatus on his face; Morrin turned him over, made a deep gash over his kidney, inserted his hand, got a hold of the ruptured kidney's pedicle and tied a ligature around it to stop the bleeding. It was over in a matter of a few minutes and long before I could administer the ether anaesthetic. The young man survived.

Whatever Morrin may have been, he was a man of quick decision and prompt action. A story is told about him that, when he was returning from a pheasant shoot in Kildare, he ran into a cow being led by his owner along the Naas road. He jumped out of the car and examined the cow, which was bellowing with pain and had obviously sustained a broken leg. He immediately took out the shotgun and shot the cow. The farmer apparently protested to Morrin about his drastic action but he stopped complaining when Morrin lifted up the shotgun and asked the man if he too was injured.

As a resident I was not infrequently instructed by him to do post-mortems on a few of his 'casualties'. He did not seek permission from the relatives, which was customary, so that the procedure was carried out generally by me at night with the aid of a student. The first such occasion was at a late hour and was an eerie experience. After attending to the front of the deceased, we turned the body over on its face and, as we did so, a long high-pitched whistling sound was emitted by the corpse as the air in the lungs was forced out through the larynx stiff with rigor mortis. On another occasion we were halfway through the procedure late at night when the relatives arrived at the locked door and demanded admission. We had to finish the job hurriedly and escape by a rear entrance.

During the years of the coronary epidemic in the 1960s and 1970s, when we were researching the nature and causes of the disease, we did a routine post-mortem examination on patients who died, always with the permission of the closest relative. It was an important exercise in learning. Our request for permission to do an autopsy was never refused as long as the approach to the request was couched in diplomatic and compassionate terms. In recent years post-mortems are rarely performed unless requested by the coroner or in the event of some unusual problem in diagnosis. Unlike more recent times, there was no problem raised to retaining the heart if we needed to carry out a careful examination of the coronary arteries and heart muscle. Times have certainly changed, as organ retention by the pathologist for further examination following the post-mortem has led to increasing concern among the public and the media.

During the summer months of July, August and September of 1945 I gave all the anaesthetics in the hospital when Morrin and Harry Meade each did a six-week stint to keep the surgical service going. I gave in excess of a hundred anaesthetics in all, becoming mildly and temporarily addicted to ether, thanks to the ease of inhaling this volatile drug through the top of the Clover apparatus. Subsequently it was suggested by one of the surgeons that I should train as an anaesthetist, presumably to return to the staff of the hospital. Fortunately, having already made up my mind to train as a cardiologist, I refused this flattering offer. Towards the end of my stay at St Vincent's, one of the younger surgeons, Paddy FitzGerald, offered me the post of surgical registrar at St Kevin's Hospital, where he also worked, but again I refused the offer, although on this occasion to refuse was more difficult because at the time I had no prospects of a post elsewhere. I mention this to underline my commitment to cardiology, a commitment which compelled me to refuse the flattering offers I had received as a resident at St Vincent's.

As a resident doctor, I lived officially in the residency of the hospital, where the food cost us twenty-five shillings each week, exactly the amount of my weekly salary! The food was unbelievably bad, even to our unsophisticated tastes, and the service from our attendant, who combined his role as housekeeper with that of sacristan, was worse. I was lucky in that my house was less than a mile away and I was constantly at Maggie's doorstep to seek extra rations and to stay nights. Maggie O'Connor was mother's newly arrived housekeeper from Wexford and was to prove a treasure to my parents during her long association with the family. Our attendant in the residency was a small, unprepossessing and sleazy character who was obsequious even to us (but whom we always suspected acted as a trusted informant on behalf of the hospital authorities).

I was appointed senior house officer to the hospital for the first six months of 1946, when again I did three months each on the medical and surgical sides. My salary was increased to thirty-two shillings and I became responsible for order and discipline in the residency, an office which I conducted with little enthusiasm and less success, and hence with no loss of my limited popularity with my peers.

On a few occasions I had a brush with the nuns about the quality of the food and the standard of service. The food was served in a sparse dining room on patterned and shredded linoleum which covered an old pine table in the old Georgian building standing between the hospital and Loreto College. Food was served strictly at the appointed hour, irrespective of our whereabouts and our clinical commitments. On one occasion

I entered our bleak and empty dining room, late for my evening meal as usual. I found a large chipped square enamel basin which contained cold sausages and coarse leaves of lettuce embedded in a semi-solid lukewarm base of discoloured lard. In a moment of fury, and throwing all discretion to the wind, I grabbed the container, carried it over to the hospital and was on my way to the mother rectress, the sole arbiter and authority of the institution, when fortunately for myself and my future career I was intercepted by Mother Canitius, the sister ministress. She dragged me into her little cubby-hole in the corridor and, with a mixture of kindness and firmness, cooled me down with honeyed words of sympathy and promises of a new and exciting cuisine. Nothing was ever done about it, but at least I can be grateful that the nuns turned a blind eye to my complaints and did not hold it against me when I returned to the consultant staff in the autumn of 1950.

Sister Canitius was one of the many grand old ladies of the Charity Order. As late as Christmas 1995 I called on her at her community home in Donnybrook. She was then ninety-four years of age, and greatly disabled physically but with a mind as clear as the day I first met her; she died in January 2000. During an animated conversation, she recalled the incident of the sausages and lard with great humour.

The bedroom I shared with three other colleagues was equally bleak and uncomfortable: it had old iron or brass bedsteads of various vintages, and cold, frayed linoleum covering the floor, and there was a large draughty Georgian window facing east. Despite the rather primitive conditions under which we lived in St Vincent's Hospital, and despite our lowly status in the scheme of things as young doctors, I recall these as very happy and carefree days. We were certainly free of any anxieties about money, for we had none; nor were we too concerned about our immediate future, being happy to have the privilege of working in St Vincent's and being still in the full flush of idealism about our chosen profession. The concept of young, recently qualified doctors having any political power or influence within the profession, as exists among the non-consultant hospital doctors today, would have been unthinkable; nor did thoughts of discrimination or hardship imposed on us by our long hours of menial work or the paucity of our remuneration ever enter our heads, apart from an occasional good-humoured grouse. I recall the great sense of fulfilment which I enjoyed when I was working as a young doctor in the hospital environment and the satisfaction derived from being part of a group of people in an institution devoted to the service of others. When I was on the resident staff of the Hospital of St John and St Elizabeth in London, I had every Thursday afternoon and evening, and every second weekend, off. These restricted hours of freedom, less generous than at St Vincent's, caused me no problems or resentment, living as I was in an institution which was fully self-contained in terms of work, social activities and human contact, and which tended to enhance one's own sense of identity and sense of purpose.

It was during the second six months of my senior residency at St Vincent's that I read the life of William Osler, the great turn-of-the-century Canadian physician. His life and essays, including his famous essay *Aequanimitas*, had a profound effect on my medical career in terms of increasing my commitment to medicine and therefore to patients' care, and also in accepting the 'slings and arrows of outrageous fortune' with equanimity. In later years and for a limited period I used to give a copy of *Aequanimitas* and other essays to every resident who joined my team at St Vincent's.

To follow a career in cardiology after leaving St Vincent's Hospital, it was necessary for me to go to England. However the summer of 1946, immediately after the war, was a time of great austerity and of severe job shortages and a scarcity of opportunities for postgraduate training because of the massive demobilisation of doctors and the preference given to those who had been in the forces. I was without a job from July to November 1946, apart from doing morning sessions at the Dublin Rheumatism Clinic, where Tom O'Reilly was the director. I was paid £1 per week. The clinic was an institution in Upper Mount Street which was established and run by the Department of Local Government and Public Health, the precursor of the Department of Health. Tom O'Reilly was a bachelor from Wexford and a staunch supporter of the Fianna Fáil anti-Treaty party, but still an old friend and admirer of my mother's. He had a thin, spare figure and an arid look about him which was consistent with his austere habits. He was soft spoken and unobtrusive in his manner, but he had a great dedication to his work, his patients and the clinic, despite the inevitable frustrations of working in an institution controlled by a parsimonious government department.

The clinic was run on a shoestring, and lacked all the equipment and facilities we expect in such institutions today, apart from a primitive physiotherapy department with mud baths and massage. Not a great deal could be done for the patients apart from them being given mild painkilling drugs and some placebo medications, but the clinic was popular and well attended because of the interest and dedication of Dr O'Reilly and his staff as well as the treatment they provided, whether it was effective or not. At least no harm was done by commission, but the effective rehabilitation techniques, which are available nowadays to patients with rheumatoid arthritis and other chronic musculo-skeletal afflictions, were not yet available. Immobilisation was still widely advised and resulted in many patients being confined to bed with contractures and deformities which were pitiful to see and which caused untold misery and severe nursing problems. Modern surgical techniques, such as joint replacement, which have been so successful, were still a long way off.

When I started in the clinic in August 1946, I suggested to the director that we should acquire erythrocyte sedimentation tubes, and a stand to hold them, to assist us in measuring the severity, the response to treatment and the prognosis of rheumatoid arthritis and other inflammatory and malignant diseases. This is a simple but useful blood test. As I recall it, the director agreed without any great conviction. I applied to the Department to purchase the equipment, the cost of which was about two shillings and sixpence. Department approval was received in November, just as I was leaving for work in England.

The Dublin Rheumatism Clinic was eventually closed by the Department of Health. It was a relic of the medicine that was practised in times when the most that could be offered to the sick was the comfort and confidence imparted by the fatherly figure of the doctor, by the caring figure of the nurse, by the penetrating odour of some exotic inhalation or application, and the colour and unpleasant taste of some arcane medicine. Since then rheumatology has become an important speciality and is a vital component of modern medicine. Great strides in treating and rehabilitating patients with the chronic rheumatic diseases have been made, although their epidemiology has so far not received sufficient attention. It is unusual now to find a patient who is totally disabled by rheumatoid arthritis, ankylosing spondylitis or osteoarthritis, thanks to modern drug and surgical treatments, physiotherapy and well-established rehabilitation procedures.

In the early forties there was little we could do to slow or halt the disease process in patients with coronary disease, stroke, high blood pressure, kidney disease, arthritis and the many bacterial and infectious conditions, such as pneumonia, meningitis and endocarditis; although by then the first antibiotics, the sulphonamides, were about to arrive. Nor could we do anything worthwhile to relieve the medical consequences of poverty and destitution. Looking further back to previous decades and centuries, there was little physicians could do to alleviate or cure except, like the clergy-man, give a sense of authority – bordering sometimes on the omniscient – which was a source of comfort and reassurance to the patient and the patient's family. In fact, when one reads of the purging, cupping, bleeding, counter-irritation, and other empirical procedures which were widely adopted in earlier centuries, one wonders if doctors did more harm than good as a result of some of their ministrations. Dogma among our medical predecessors varied in direct proportion to their incompetence or igno-rance – a human weakness which has not yet passed into history in our profession.

Not all of these strictures apply to surgery in the early 1940s. Although surgical morbidity and mortality were high, at least some operations served to help or cure patients, and to return them to a normal life. However, the fashionable, unproven, useless and possibly harmful opera-tions, which have been a feature of surgical practice since records began, were widespread, just as many medical treatments, such as those described in the previous paragraph, have never been validated and can have done nothing but harm. The operations which were widely adopted during my early years and were subsequently shown to be useless or harmful are too numerous to be listed here: tonsillectomy, circumcision, sympathectomy for high blood pressure and leg vessel disease, and numerous abdominal and gynaecological procedures. As a senior resident I gave anaesthetics for a dentist who carried out total dental extractions at the request of physicians who believed the teeth were the source of some unexplained infections. Even among the young the teeth were extracted without research evidence to justify such a procedure. Surgery of the nasal sinuses was not infrequently carried out in patients with nasal catarrh and are now rarely performed or thought necessary.

There are lessons to be learnt in the new millennium from medical practice during the nineteenth and early twentieth centuries. We achieve cure in many more cases now but at a price which is considerable, if difficult to measure. Our interventions are more complicated, and at times more dangerous, and more expensive. The great technical advances made in diagnosis and treatment, and the wide variety of potent drugs available, may have outstripped the judgement and training of some doctors. The increasing ability to keep patients alive, even those with an unacceptable quality of life, and the commercialisation of medicine, have created major ethical problems for doctors and medical institutions.

The sick must be treated, but it is useful to remind ourselves of the vast sums of money spent in western countries on their treatment as part of the ironically named 'health services', with little or no impact on the public health or on life expectation. By their very nature, the chronic non-communicable diseases which afflict modern western society will only respond to prevention and to appropriate changes in lifestyle and our environment. We can at least take personal control of our health nowadays, thanks to the gradual discovery of the causes of chronic disease; the increasing awareness and advocacy of public health measures, better general education and the elimination of the diseases of contagion and infection which were rampant in the past and beyond our personal control.

3

POSTGRADUATE TRAINING IN POST-WAR LONDON

In November 1946 I obtained a one-month locum as a house physician at the Hospital of St John and St Elizabeth, a voluntary hospital in St John's Wood. Administered by the Sisters of Mercy, it was closely associated with the diocese of Westminster and its cardinal archbishop. The medical staff mostly reflected its Catholic ethos, although a few physicians there were non-Catholic. It was a relatively small hospital with an elitist reputation because of its association with the diocese, its distinguished medical staff drawn from Harley Street and the London teaching hospitals, its well-regarded nursing school, its special facilities for private patients, and its location in an upmarket inner suburb of London.

I was subsequently appointed as a house physician for a year, during which I continued to live in and enjoy the friendly and happy atmosphere of the staff and surroundings of the hospital. I was then the lone house physician in a hospital of about 140 beds, and without a senior resident I found myself responsible for all the medical patients under the care of the various attending physicians. I was paid the princely sum of £100 per year, but this did not worry me too much although my social life was still greatly restricted by a chronic lack of money. During my first two years in

London I had little contact with English society outside the hospital and remained only vaguely conscious that I was in a foreign land and living in a different culture than my own. It was a measure of my immaturity. This outlook was perpetuated by my contact with the Irish University Club and my frequent visits to Irish families. Some of the Irish I met in the club seemed to live in a fantasy world: constantly aware of their origins and proclaiming nostalgia for Ireland and, in social terms at least, remaining resolutely outside the English social scene. The University Club was popular, particularly for those with a National University of Ireland background. Its members were, as far as I can recall, all Irish immigrants or birds of passage, and its ambience was that of the gregariousness and love of *craic* of the Irish. Drink was an important binding factor in an environment befogged by the ubiquitous cigarette. We were all smokers in the late forties as the supply of cigarettes improved after the shortages of the war.

When I later spent more time with English or Anglo-Irish families whom I met or for whom I worked, I found that their culture and mores differed little from those in Ireland. I was impressed by the fairness and the integrity of the British, and by their commitment to the law, even in matters about which we in Ireland appear to have a more casual concern. Our neutrality during the war seemed of little interest to the British and was never referred to in my contact with the Londoners.

I enjoyed my four years in London and admired the English for their hospitality, their tolerance and their fondness for the Irish; the only exceptions were a few clerics attached to the Diocese of Westminster. I felt they were less tolerant of the Catholics in England who identified with the Irish Diaspora. This was particularly well illustrated by the service I attended at Westminster Cathedral on the occasion of the celebration of the four hundredth anniversary of the martyrdom of Sir Thomas More. A comfortably padded monsignor spoke with great eloquence to the title 'The Revival of Catholicism in England'. His lengthy sermon described the roots and evolution of English Catholicism, particularly during the early part of the nineteenth century. He made little reference to the huge Irish Diaspora and its contribution to English Catholicism. I was sometimes conscious of the patronising attitude of some of these Westminster clerics I was introduced to, some of whom we addressed as 'monsignor'. All seemed well dressed and shod, portly and self-satisfied. They appeared to find the principal pleasure in life at the dining table, apart from whatever functions they employed and spiritual graces they enjoyed. My only contact with the Cardinal Archbishop was my duty in carrying his train into the hospital's chapel on one of his official visits.

At the end of my year as a resident, the hospital created the part-time post of medical registrar for me. This allowed me to start training as a cardiologist at the National Heart Hospital and to prepare for the College of Physicians membership examination. I was now paid £200 per year, living outside the hospital, and my digs in Miss Galvin's at St John's Wood High Street became my home for the rest of my stay in London. Miss Galvin was a gentle, kindly creature who did her best to make my life comfortable and homely, despite the dowdy bedroom I occupied. She was of Irish origin and had a soft spot for the young Irish doctors, who were glad of her lodgings and who succeeded me at St John and St Elizabeth's. Jack Flanagan of Swords, County Dublin, and later of St Kevin's Hospital, preceded me at the hospital; others to follow were Joe McMullin and Dermot Cantwell, both of whom, like myself, were students at St Vincent's Hospital and were subsequently appointed to the staff of St Vincent's. Many hospitals in England had the same experience as mine at St John and St Elizabeth's: once an Irish graduate had joined the resident staff, he or she was followed by a succession of Irish graduates – surely a tribute to our chauvinism and a measure of confidence in us shown by our English hosts. Rita Clery, from the Kerry Gaelteacht, who had been one of our Irish-speaking governesses in Lissenfield in the early 1930s, was the radiographer at the hospital when I arrived. Rita and I occasionally spoke Irish to puzzle English fellow passengers in the underground. She was replaced by Barbara Foley, a tall, handsome and comely girl whose company I enjoyed, although in an entirely platonic way. Barbara married Niall St John McCarthy, who became a distinguished judge of the Supreme Court in Ireland. They both died tragically in a road traffic accident in Spain in 1992.

Two years at St John and St Elizabeth's had a powerful effect on my future medical career, mainly because of the influence of two physicians, Hugh Dunlop and Pat Corridan. As house physician and subsequently registrar, I worked closely with them and with another physician (who lacked their clinical skills). When I left Dublin I was poorly equipped in the art and science of internal medicine. I had little insight into the diagnosis of disease and the understanding of patients' problems which comes with that subtle association and interaction of symptoms, physical signs, and knowledge of anatomy, physiology and pathology. These are the components which provide the elements of the final clinical presentation, and without them it is impossible to gain an insight into the physical and mental processes that constitute disease.

I was soon to be reminded of my clinical ignorance when, shortly after my appointment, I sent urgently for the neurologist, who was on emergency duty late at night. A patient had suddenly become breathless and distressed. The neurologist arrived, made a very cursory examination and turned scathingly to me and asked why, if it was a true emergency, did the patient had a normal colour. It was in fact a hysterical attack, and it was clearly obvious to him that it had no organic origin. I was not likely to make the same error of judgement again.

My contact with Dunlop and Corridan, and the easy access at that time to various clinical teaching sessions in other London teaching hospitals, soon gave me an insight which I had theretofore lacked of the fundamentals of history-taking and bedside examination. I realised how inadequate my training had been. Both Dunlop and Corridan earned my admiration and gratitude because of their methodical approach to every patient through careful history-taking and physical examination, their expert reliance on classical clinical methods and their obvious care and concern for their patients. I found myself developing new skills of diagnosis and management by embracing their good example and teaching skills. The exercise of diagnosis was challenging and exciting, in the same way that the reader enjoys unravelling the problems posed by Agatha Christie in her classic detective novels. During my four years in London I acquired an increasing interest in people and a curiosity about their problems, whether psychological, social or medical, which made medical practice an absorbing and satisfying lifetime occupation.

Dunlop was a bachelor and a delightfully benign eccentric whose whole life was devoted to his professional work and to teaching. He was on the medical staff of the Charing Cross Hospital, where many of the consultants were women. He had a booming voice and a refreshing frankness. On one occasion at the bedside of a patient whom he had discharged home, the patient asked Dunlop if he would prescribe him an aphrodisiac. He replied in his booming voice for all in the ward to hear, 'The best aphrodisiac is the inside of a woman's thigh'! Surely remarkable insight for a confirmed bachelor!

Corridan, who was a Catholic and also a bachelor, had qualified in University College Cork. He had close contact with the Westminster clergy and was appointed physician to the Cardinal Archbishop. He had all the qualities of a good doctor. Corridan unfortunately smoked heavily and died suddenly in his forties. In the late 1940s there was little suspicion of the close relationship between cigarette smoking, coronary heart disease and sudden, unexpected death.

The third physician with whom I worked was in striking contrast with his two colleagues in his casual approach to clinical methods. He would have been described in popular parlance as eminent, although the competence of such members of my profession may be in inverse proportion to their public recognition. He was physician to the Royal Household and was later to be physician to King George VI – and to become noteworthy for missing the King's lung cancer, and sending him with his 'touch of pneumonitis' to Balmoral to convalesce. He was the quintessential Harley Street physician: fashionable, dogmatic, patronising and overly ambitious, the master of the snap diagnosis based on inspired guesswork rather than careful and systematic enquiry. I think I learned as much from him as I did from Corridan and Dunlop, if only because he taught me the pitfalls of neglecting the well-established principles of medical diagnosis and of failing to admit one's own ignorance or uncertainty. Two years with Corridan and Dunlop advanced my knowledge of medical practice, and confirmed a resolution never to accept responsibility for a patient's wellbeing without personally making or confirming the diagnosis, and that I would always acknowledge my own ignorance or uncertainty if ever encountered.

However, the physician to the Royal Household was not without wit and charm, combined with a little cynicism. On one occasion he observed a Catholic patient receiving the last rites of the Church before undergoing a major operation. While he was waiting to speak to the surgeon, he enquired of me the nature of the ceremony. He was of course well aware of the Catholic ethos of the hospital. I explained that it was a sacrament of the Church which was administered to those who are in danger of dying and that it confers an added grace when one arrives in the next world. He replied that it would surely upset the patient if he or she were aware of their imminent demise. 'On the contrary,' I said, 'it often reassures the patient to know that they have received such a blessing from God through the hands of a priest.' I added, 'And the confidence the sacrament inspires in the faithful may well contribute to the patient's recovery!' This information was received by him with apparent interest and, following a thoughtful moment, he addressed me in a most serious tone saying, 'Should we not therefore add extreme unction to the pharmacopeia?'

Despite his shortcomings as a physician, he was a gracious colleague and a pleasure to work with. Notwithstanding his seniority and his patrician background, he did become a friend of mine and I enjoyed the hospitality of his house and home in Harley Street. The worst time in terms of food shortage in London was 1946–47. I arranged several visits for him and his wife to visit Dublin at weekends, to stay in the Russell Hotel and to shower hospitality on my parents at Jammet's restaurant. He returned to London and the hospital in high good humour after consuming a few fillet steaks, which he described as *au point*. He was also intrigued by making the acquaintance of my father, the man who led the War of Independence against his country. I often wonder if I had married one of his daughters, both of whom I knew, would I have become physician to the queen, or at least to her household? I now regret that I did not think of such an enterprise. He was Welsh and might not have objected to his daughter marrying a Catholic, although the queen might not have been so tolerant. With my likely influence at the palace, perhaps the Good Friday agreement might have been reached earlier!

St John and St Elizabeth's had a strong, charitable and Irish ethos provided by the presence of the Sisters of Mercy, who owned the hospital. Its nursing school was highly thought of and was much sought after by students from Ireland and Wales. It was for me an enjoyable and productive time, thanks to my being the sole resident on the medical side, I was not adversely affected by the austerities, the monotonous diet of whale and horse meat, the Yorkshire pudding-like substitute for potatoes and the absence of any variety in the cuisine. Cigarettes were hard to find, and often only by including the publican in one of your rounds of drink.

Unlike the Irish publicans, many of whom were teetotallers, the innkeepers of England were not reluctant to join their customers in their habits. After all, was it not Omar Khayyam who wondered, 'why not'?

The British National Health Service was established by Aneuryn Bevan and the Labour government in 1948 while I was in London. It was a time of great ferment within the medical profession, whose representatives were largely opposed to the measure, although it mattered little to me and other postgraduate students. Cardinal Griffin refused to allow St John and St Elizabeth's to join the new service. This appeared to be a critical decision which caused uncertainty about the hospital's future. Nevertheless, it became a successful private hospital which prospered because of the increasing numbers of citizens who had access to private health insurance.

During my three years as a postdoctoral student at the National Heart Hospital, I encountered physicians who were excellent clinicians. It was before the era of high technology in cardiac practice: they relied largely on their senses to achieve a high degree of diagnostic accuracy. Great progress was being made by them in the clinical diagnosis of heart disease and particularly congenital and valve disease, thanks to insights provided by catheter studies and the application of catheter findings to clinical signs. Some of the great pioneers during that period worked in the National Heart Hospital. I had the impression during my time there that great things were happening in the field of heart disease research and progress, particularly in sharpening bedside diagnosis.

My visits to the National Hospital for Nervous Diseases in Queen Square were also inspirational because of the fine tradition of teaching and practice there, as were my attendances at the Middlesex with Dr Beaumont, at the London Hospital with Dr Donald Hunter and Dr Denis Williams at George's. These were the days when the London teaching hospitals reached the peak of their fame, which they earned because of the high standards set by many of their consultant staffs. Clinical teaching excelled in these London teaching hospitals and, like other postgraduate students, I was free to attend all their teaching sessions. The consultants I encountered were devoted to their teaching and were gracious in dealing with callow young postgraduate doctors eager to learn and to prepare for the entrance exam to membership of the Royal College of Physicians.

My first visit to one of these great institutions was to the Middlesex Hospital, where Dr Beaumont held a session every Wednesday morning. He was the author of a textbook on medicine which was the standard work we used as undergraduates in Dublin. I introduced myself to the sister who was to accompany Dr Beaumont on his teaching round. She informed him that I wished to attend and that I had qualified in Dublin. As soon as he and about thirty other postgraduates had gathered around the first patient, I was thrown into the deep end by his asking for the young doctor from Dublin. He shook my hand and then asked me to seek a history from the incumbent in the bed. Being unused to such prominence, particularly in strange surroundings and with a formidable audience, I was nearly struck dumb; but his patience and reassuring presence allowed me to recover and to proceed with my history-taking, after which I was required to examine the patient. He was constructively critical and was diplomatic in pointing to my shortcomings, although he added a reassuring note about my possible future as a clinician.

It was my many visits to the London teaching hospitals and my custom of carrying a textbook of medicine with me on my many bus and underground journeys that accounts for my successfully passing the examination for membership of the Royal College of Physicians within eighteen months of my arrival in London. This was a prestigious postgraduate achievement at the time and did not go unnoticed by my teachers at St Vincent's Hospital.

London after the war was a drab place. No fresh coat of paint was to be seen; indeed it was many years before the buildings and the many terraces of houses were restored to their former freshness and brightness. Bomb-sites and derelict buildings were scattered everywhere. Despite these signs and scars of war, and the austerity, which was at its most extreme in the late forties, London was a most pleasant place to live in – at least in upmarket St John's Wood, and in the central part of the metropolis. The local services were excellent, and much better apparently than they are today. Travel on buses and the underground was cheap and efficient, the people were no different in manners and behaviour from those in Dublin, and security day or night was absolute, and was personified by the presence and popularity of the London bobby.

Medicine is described as a vocation based on art and science: without both, it cannot serve its function in helping the sick. With the exception of some surgical operations and limited areas in medicine, such as the management of diabetes, it was almost entirely an art up to the time of the Second World War. Bedside manner might have been its most important component. It was only then and afterwards that the scientific approach to medicine arrived, with its emphasis on accurate diagnosis and evidence-based treatments provided by clinical trials assisted by new investigative procedures and post-mortem studies. It was in the Heart Hospital and in a few centres in America that, for the first time, the definition and diagnosis of most heart abnormalities were established through the correlation of clinical signs and symptoms with the underlying structural defects and muscular changes in the heart and its blood vessels.

The National Heart Hospital was staffed by specialist physicians who had the advantage of close contact with each other and who shared an interest in clinical research, treatment and teaching and whose work was to bring great benefit to other institutions throughout the world. I never gained an official residency appointment at the National Heart Hospital or other London teaching hospitals. This was again because of the many doctors who had been discharged from the forces and who were seeking training opportunities in the specialist and teaching hospitals. I could come and go as I pleased despite my non-residency status and in many ways I benefited by being in attendance during the ward rounds and out-patient sessions of all the consultants and without the routine chores of the residents. From the aspect of clinical bedside medicine, my training proved to be ideal.

I did mature in a number of ways during my four years in London. My commitment to the more secular aspects of Catholicism largely evaporated. My first wife had lapsed before I met her. However, I continued to attend Sunday mass while I lived with my parents, and later when my children were growing up. I did not wish to cause any upset to my parents, nor did I want my girls and boys, who were attending Catholic primary schools, to find themselves in an anomalous position with their teachers and their peers because their dad did not go to mass.

To move to lighter things, early in January 1947, shortly after I had arrived in London, I was confined to bed in the residency with a bad bout of influenza. It had been snowing heavily and the weather had been bitterly cold. Quite unexpectedly, Kevin O'Sullivan arrived into my bedroom. He was one of my closest associates in the UCD Boat Club, where he, Des Hogan and I formed a loose triumvirate. I was delighted to see him, being still a little homesick and naturally somewhat depressed by the flu virus. He brought a gift of a bottle of Power's Gold Label whiskey, a beverage which was hardly available in England at that time. I insisted that we should share a glass on that cold inclement night. Its effect was to increase the warmth of our reunion and to replace my viral ennui by a welcome feeling of euphoria. We finished the bottle and, as one might anticipate, thanks to my illness and to my empty stomach, I was in an advanced state of inebriation by then. I led Kevin through the hospital corridors in my dressing gown; we left by the back entrance and I accompanied him a distance of about three hundred yards through the packed snow and slush to see him on to the last Bakerloo train from St John's Wood station. I was accosted by an off-duty hospital porter when we arrived at the railway station, and discreetly led back to my room. Next day, despite a hangover, I was able to return to my normal duties in the hospital. This episode was my first clue to the value of Irish whiskey: that if taken in adequate amounts, it is an effective antidote to the virus of influenza and the common cold.

On another occasion, on one of the days of my afternoon and evening off, I was given two free tickets to attend a London theatre that evening. Free theatre tickets were frequently made available at short notice to hospital staff when the shows were not fully booked. I contacted another rowing colleague who was doing a general-practice locum in Hampstead Heath nearby. He was a teetotaller during his years in college, but a few years knocking around England doing locums and visiting Irish clubs had changed his habits. He was now an episodic drinker with a tendency to *mania a potu*, a form of acute mania induced by alcohol. My invitation to him proved to be unfortunate. He picked me up in his battered old Rover. Because we found the first act of the vapid upper-middle-class English comedy to be boring and tedious, we retired to the bar for the rest of the performance. We stayed there until the theatre closed and then retired to the Captain's Cabin, a well-known underground pub in Piccadilly. Here we continued to imbibe until our money ran out; we then went off then to the University Club in Victoria, where our credit was good and the drink was plentiful.

My companion became extremely drunk and bellicose, and despite many entreaties insisted on driving home. I was hardly sober myself, but I had enough savvy to know that he was incapable of driving, and I felt apprehensive about going with him. However, whether it was through loyalty to him or because of his insistence, I found myself being driven at breakneck speed from the club up to Hyde Park Corner, where he crashed into the back of a red post office van. Reversing quickly, he made a sharp turn and drove straight across the street into Hyde Park. At this stage I remembered no more until I found myself being removed from the car and bundled into a large black van by a few policemen. We had apparently crashed through the barrier of a building site and finished up embedded in a heap of sand. I spent the night in a cell in Hampstead Heath police station, aware of my friend in the next cell ranting and shouting invective at the police about the injustices in the North of Ireland.

Early that morning I was put back in the Black Maria and returned to the hospital. Unfortunately, instead of dumping me at the more discreet and unobtrusive back entrance to the hospital, the Black Maria drove through the imposing front gates into the large quadrangle in front. On the right was the nurses' home, on the left the convent, and between it and the hospital, the chapel. As I was let out of the van, a procession of nuns was proceeding from the convent to the chapel to attend seven o'clock mass. My appearance, accompanied by the police officers, must have greatly shocked the poor nuns.

I had been appointed medical registrar a few days before but on the afternoon of my conspicuous appearance in the quadrangle I was interviewed by the chairman of the medical board and advised that I was now deemed unsuitable for such a responsible position. I was coming to the end of my year as house physician and now found myself without the prospect of immediate employment. However, the day was saved because the 'also-rans' who had unsuccessfully applied for the post were no longer available. The hospital had no choice but to take me, despite my recently acquired reputation of being an alcoholic and a lawbreaker to wit. My erring companion was discreetly returned to his house and surgery in the morning. No action was taken against him despite the provocation the police must have endured listening to his political ranting, nor was anything ever heard about the post office van. It was another example of the tolerance the English bobby showed to the many Irish doctors who were practising in England at that time, and who might have had a weakness for the little drop!

Such exploits were fortunately rare events, but I did have another outing with the same person and two other rowing friends. The four of us met at Marble Arch at midday on the Saturday of the August bank holiday. The driver, like the other two, was a general practitioner. He was driving a large and ancient Triumph as we set off for Brighton for the weekend. We had a few stops at public houses during our journey, and did not arrive in Brighton until midnight. By this time we were in euphoric mood. We could find no place to stay, nor could we find any night spots to continue our carousing. We had no alternative but to sleep rough, but the south coast of England in the Brighton region was even then a vast conurbation and provided few places where we could stretch out for the night. We drove westwards along the coast for a considerable length of time but eventually in the darkness we found a patch of grass beside the road where we settled for the remainder of the night. I slept in the front of the car, a companion in the back, while the other two stretched out on the green sward beside the car.

I was wakened in the early morning by a frightful din. We had driven on to the immaculate lawn of a large hotel in Littlehampton, one of the upmarket resorts on the south coast. We were surrounded by flower beds and shrubberies and in the distance there was a model railway for children. About one hundred yards ahead of us was a huge and imposing emporium. The din was caused by my two companions outside being harangued and accosted by two or three liveried staff who were enraged by our trespass. Our driver, who had been captain of the Boat Club in my time, was known for his prompt decision-making and firm leadership. He and his sleeping partner took the only sensible action that was feasible on this embarrassing occasion: they jumped straight into the car and we sped away – the makers of the Triumph would have been proud of the car's remarkable ten-second acceleration from the starting position.

Our next stop was Bognor Regis where, due to my hangover and to the fact that I had exhausted my money, I thankfully got on the first train I could catch and returned to the hospital to recuperate. I was fortunate then and since that these exploits were unusual events. I could never take part in a drinking spree over any long period of time, because of a reactive depression which invariably set in and which acted as a most effective antidote to the desire to continue drinking. Part of the depression was the sense of guilt at harming my physical integrity, my mental faculties, and my self-esteem.

After the Royal College of Physicians membership examination had been passed I spent spare time from the Heart Hospital doing general-practice locum work, particularly for the Carey family in Lewisham. They had come from Killarney in County Kerry and were well established in this inner London suburb. I was obliged to do night surgeries elsewhere in London to supplement my meagre honorarium as a part-time registrar at St John and St Elizabeth's Hospital, and later as an unpaid full-time post-graduate student at the Heart Hospital. I would go by Underground to surgeries in Lewisham, Sidcup, Ruislip, Ealing, North Finchley or some other godforsaken outer suburb. I had a good capacity to read, write and concentrate while travelling, and later in my career I put this gift to good use when writing research articles and health-promotion literature during my worldwide travels to research centres.

The London suburbs had a dull uniformity about them just after the war, accentuated by the absence of paint and colour. I seldom met the principal of the night surgery, except when I stayed with families. I would be admitted by a caretaker or housekeeper, who would be my only contact. Hiring locums to do night surgeries became a widespread feature of the new NHS after it was established by Aneuryn Bevan and the post-war socialist government in 1948.

The surgeries were crowded, and the service given by locum doctors must have been unsatisfactory, but perhaps no worse than that demanded by a passive British public. It was impossible to practise medicine according to the precepts of our teachers and our teaching hospitals because of the numbers of patients attending, the poor facilities available to examine patients and the traditional acceptance by both patient and doctor of a consultation that usually lasted only as long as was necessary to write out a prescription. I was soon to learn that the keystone of modern and orthodox medicine, at least at the general practice level, was the ritual of prescribing a medicine. At least writing the prescription takes less time than the shortest conversation or words of reassurance.

Counselling played little part in the practices I encountered. Many of the patients attending these surgeries needed a repeat prescription or a certificate of incapacity to work; many too suffered from mood problems, such as chronic depression or loneliness, or were victims of poor social circumstances or of chronic, disturbed personal relationships. They needed counselling and social support, not a bottle of medicine; but because of the restraints of time and the under-funding of the services, and because doctors are not often trained in the art of counselling, the ritual of routine prescribing was the rule.

The first surgery I attended was in Sidcup. There were many doctors from Ireland in practice in England at that time and this practice was run by two brothers from Cork. I never met the two principals in my visits to their surgery; I was met by the housekeeper and was put straight to work. There must have been about forty patients waiting on my first visit. In my innocence, I attempted to take a history from each, finding that the cryptic and illegible notes which the practitioners were obliged to keep under the terms of their contract were quite useless. I also attempted to examine some of the patients. One particular patient, a diminutive old lady in a long heavy black frieze coat, was obviously suffering from chronic asthma. She attended the surgery regularly to collect her prescription for a cough medicine and ephedrine tablets. She must have been surprised when I refused to write her a prescription without examining her first. She resisted but, eventually, agreed to open the upper button of her overcoat. Through a small aperture over her breast bone I managed to insert the chest piece of my stethoscope. As I listened to the cacophony of her wheezing breath, she looked at me benignly, smiled and said in her cockney accent, 'I suppose that, when you have the same experience as Dr Murphy, you'll be able to hear through my overcoat too!'

That particular night I was proceeding so slowly that the housekeeper had to intervene to remind me that the last train left for Baker Street at such an hour and that I was likely to miss it. The rest of the surgery was conducted along more practical and traditional lines.

I very quickly got into the routine of general practice, and became quite proficient in dealing expeditiously with large numbers of patients. It was clearly impossible to fight the system and I was sufficiently pragmatic to adjust to it without delay or any misgivings. In fact, the great bulk of the patients were chronic attendees who appeared to be satisfied with the transitory contact with their doctor. The medicine bottle was the bond that united them and the doctor might have been the symbol of their father figure. It was more a social than a medical service, particularly as most of the medicines prescribed were placebos and had no proven therapeutic value. At least, unlike many of the drugs in the modern pharmacopoeia, the medicines in the late forties did not have the same potential to do harm, nor were they the same drain on the public purse. The regular visit to the doctor might have been an alternative to the confessional, which was a regular and obligatory practice for Roman Catholics. The Roman Catholic priests, as they became depleted in numbers and occupied by other responsibilities, were able to dispense with the confessional. Hopefully the modern health service in the UK has eliminated the overcrowded general practice surgery and the overcrowded outpatient departments which prevailed in London in the 1940s.

I should make it clear that the above remarks about general practice refer specifically to the service I encountered in some suburban areas in London in the late 1940s. It was the same in other British cities and perhaps parts of the Irish urban scene as well. Many aspects of general practice were different in rural and in upper class urban areas, where the overcrowding and demeaning impersonal contact between patient and doctor was less evident.

Any problem which could not be dealt with at general practice level was referred to the local hospital with a hurried note saying 'Please see' or, in the case of the more prolix, 'Please see and advise'. The rare patient suspected of having an immediate and urgent problem was packed off directly to the hospital. Such a patient would not usually have been a regular attendee, and would be complaining of some unexpected or clearly organic symptom, such as abdominal pain or unusually severe headache. One very quickly learned to separate the wheat from the chaff, and mistakes were only made under these circumstances by lack of experience or, more often, by being in a hurry or through carelessness. Lack of experience tended to make one more cautious and therefore less likely to make mistakes.

On one occasion I saw a patient at a surgery in North Finchley, where I made a confident diagnosis of an atrial septal defect. This is a condition where there is a wide and abnormal communication between the two atria (the upper chambers of the heart). It is congenital in origin and leads to the useless partial recycling of blood within the heart. The diagnosis can be established by inspecting and feeling the chest wall, and by detecting certain murmurs and changes in the heart sounds with the stethoscope. Although the diagnosis was obvious to me following my training at the Heart Hospital, it would not be within the competence of the general practitioner to make. Indeed, most doctors would have been unaware of such an abnormality of the heart during these earlier times.

I wrote a letter with my usual almost illegible signature and referred the patient to Dr William Evans at the National Heart Hospital out-patient department, which I attended regularly. Dr Evans was a rather eccentric, larger-than-life individual, who was popular as a teacher and as a character. He, like all the doctors I encountered at the Heart Hospital, was an excellent clinician. The patient arrived a few weeks later and one can easily imagine the surprise expressed by Dr Evans and his large group of acolytes when a mere GP referred in a patient with a cryptic note asking the consultant to recommend management for his patient with an atrial septal defect! Needless to say, I stayed in the background among the gathering of residents and postgraduates to avoid being seen by the patient. It was kind of Dr Evans to write back to the doctor at North Finchley to congratulate him on the accuracy of his diagnosis!

My rather unorthodox postgraduate years in London were hugely important because of the fine mix of experience I had of all levels of practice. I also enjoyed the wider and more acceptable aspects of the service when, in my later years in London, I acted as a locum for doctors who were on holidays or indisposed. My experience, as mentioned earlier, was mainly with the Carey family in Lewisham, a less remote suburb in south London. Edward was the senior partner, and was joined by his brother, Charles, and another Irish graduate, Tom Tangney from Cork. Despite their years in London, they spoke with the rich, unadulterated accents of west Munster men. Edward had settled in London in the early twenties and later brought his brother over to join him. They and Tom Tangney provided an excellent service in the Lewisham area and were highly regarded in the neighbourhood. Irish doctors were popular in Britain because of their reputation of informality and friendliness. They lacked the formal professionalism that was part of the British doctor's veneer, although I am sure there are many exceptions to this generalisation.

Edward, who was married to an Irishwoman and whose three sons were contemporaries of mine in the medical faculty at University College Dublin, was well known in Catholic circles in London, as was Tom Tangney. Tom was also married to an Irishwoman, a Miss Hyland, who qualified as a doctor with me at UCD. Tom had a great brash personality, and a powerful and trenchant Cork accent, being a most gregarious and popular person with his wide circle of Irish friends and his English patients. Both he and Edward must have had a powerful influence on their patients because of their brisk, businesslike and outgoing personalities, and their well-developed communication skills. They were splendid ambassadors for Ireland, even if their contact was mainly with the plain people of their adopted country.

Charlie, whose family I usually stayed with, was very different. He possessed a gentle and amiable disposition, was always unhurried, retained a quiet Kerry burr, and lacked all of the bustling features of the busy general practitioner. He and his charming English wife Clare were little involved in the social scene of the Irish Diaspora. They were a delightful couple, and had six attractive teenage children. They and their children brought me for the first time into contact with the English middle class. I was impressed by their openly affectionate attitude towards each other, by their lack of inhibitions in showing their affection, and the openness and frankness of their conversation on all domestic and personal matters, including those more intimate subjects which would never be discussed in my own home in Dublin.

It was in their house that I first learned the importance of treating children as adults, even at an early age. This approach was achieved by Charlie and Clare mainly by avoiding the patronising attitude adopted by many parents to their children, and both were invariably addressed by their first names by the children. My infatuation with the Carey family was based on Charlie's gentleness and modesty, on Clare's intelligence and affectionate nature, on their children's maturity, and on the liberal relations and openness which they shared. It was with them that I experienced my first stirrings of falling in love, as I did with their daughter Ann; but she was only sixteen years and I, being foolish, thought myself too old at twenty-six.

Charlie Carey was a heavy smoker, as were his two partners, including Edward who died from emphysema before the age of seventy. From being a common and very distressing disease then, severe emphysema is now extremely rare, like the rest of the smoking-related diseases. Charlie smoked forty Churchman cigarettes daily. Even as early as the late forties, I was aware of the health hazards of smoking. I recall convincing him that his heavy smoking put him at high risk, and, much to his wife's relief and joy, he managed to quit the habit before I returned to Ireland. His partner, Tom Tangney, was also a heavy smoker, but managed to stop some time afterwards.

My participation in general practice in London was a valuable experience, not only as part of my training in medicine, but also in giving me a rich insight into medical practice and the problems and circumstances facing doctors and patients in that country. It also taught me something about the humanity and fallibility of doctors, about their altruism, about the fulfilment which could coexist with boredom and hardship, and it taught me about the quiet resignation of patients who managed, despite the shortcomings of the health service and the brief and impersonal contact with its servants, to hold their doctors in special regard

It was a measure of my immaturity that my mind was set on getting back to Dublin as soon as possible, although I should have known that the whole world was my oyster at this fertile time in the evolution of cardiology. I had decided to go to Boston for further training but my plans were interrupted by being offered a place at St Vincent's in September 1950. I had also arranged to act as a ship's doctor on a South American route but I reneged on this plan when I got the invitation to return to Dublin. Afterwards I greatly regretted my haste in returning so precipitously to my alma mater.

At that time mistakes were made by doctors but they were either unknown to the patient or, if known, were accepted with quiet resignation. Today mistakes are still being made because medicine is an art as well as a science. Art will always play a part in medicine because medical practice cannot be based exclusively on the precision of science and the scientific method. Differences in the approach to the patient and to judgement, opinions and knowledge exist among doctors and the multitude of clinical circumstances makes it inevitable that mistakes will be made, even among the most knowledgeable and conscientious. Today there is a public attitude that the errant doctor or the institution should be the object of blame and litigation. Affected patients complain to the health authorities, to the popular press, to Joe Duffy and his media colleagues, or to the local TD or counsellor. Media publicity and intrusion play a large part in a trend that is slowly damaging the relationship between the profession and the public, and is more than damaging to professional practice in terms of overuse of expensive tests, the burgeoning cost of the health services in the western world and, perhaps most serious, a blurring of the vocational traditions of my profession. Patient discontent, whether justified or not, should be treated confidentially by plaintiff and defendant, as in medical practice, and should be dealt with by an appropriate system or commission, along the lines of our ombudsmen, at least before proceeding to the law courts. Gross negligence should be treated as culpable, but should €4.5 million be awarded to parents if, largely through the vagaries of nature, their child is born with a congenital abnormality? Such tragedies should be the responsibility of the social services and the State.

My experience of general practice also extended to one period of three weeks in Ireland. I had a month without any commitments in the summer of 1949. I thought I might add to my depleted finances by doing a locum in general practice in Ireland, while at the same time making welcome contact with home and the family. I was paid seven pounds a week for my services to the dispensary (publicly assisted) patients. This was exactly what I paid for my weekly board and lodging at a small and modest hostelry and pub on the rather unkempt, narrow, long and winding main street of the small village in the heart of Munster. However, I was entitled to keep any private fees I might earn.

The principal whose locum I was doing had retired from the Irish army after the Second World War, or the Emergency as it was known in Ireland. He apparently had little experience or knowledge of general practice, but it was government policy at the time to appoint those doctors who had joined the army during the Emergency to a dispensary to ensure that they were not disadvantaged by their courage and patriotism. The doctor appointed failed to gain the confidence of the local community, apparently because of a serious error of medical judgement soon after his arrival.

The doctor's practice was largely confined to his dispensary patients. His potential private patients were attending other doctors in the surrounding towns and villages. He had no private patients, at least not for the first two weeks of my three-week stay. My dispensary duties were largely confined to handing out packets of DDT powder to those who arrived at the rather primitive and mean dispensary building.

I did, however, have one private patient during my first week. I was approached one day in the main street by a tall, gaunt, cadaverous man with a shifty look and an old cap drawn down over his eyes. Furtively looking around the street, he asked me if I was the new doctor from London. He thought he was going deaf and asked could I do something to help him. I told him to accompany me to the surgery where I could examine him. Although I was perfectly aware of the diagnosis as soon as I had a superficial look at him (because I could see the wax protruding from his two ears), I made a little fuss about examining each ear with my auriscope, and then saying, 'You've got wax in your ears. It's blocking the ear passages. I'll have to syringe them out. That should put things right.' 'And how much will that cost, doctor?' says he.

Never having discussed or been asked for a fee before, I was immediately thrown into a state of confusion, but I managed to blurt out 'a pound' and then I made the first commercial mistake of my career, although by no means my last. I added 'Ten shillings an ear!' He said, 'Well, doctor, I'll have to think about it,' and out he went to the street, no doubt to commune with his long dead mother or his favourite saint. Ten minutes later, during which time I waited with some little trepidation, he returned. 'I'll let you do one ear,' he said, 'and if that's better, sure I'll let you do the other.' So I syringed out one ear, and had my first experience of an ethical dilemma: should I do the other ear? I decided no, but I was left with a slightly uneasy feeling that Hippocrates might have disapproved.

During the next fifteen or sixteen days, I met him daily on the main street. Seeing me, he would cross to the other side of the street, pull the cap down further over his eyes, and pass me by, no doubt certain that I would not recognise him. I never heard what happened to his second ear, but he will remain forever in my memory as the first patient to pay me a private fee. Incidentally, my first private fee as a consultant was earned in October 1950, just after I had returned to St Vincent's Hospital. A farmer arrived in from Tipperary and as he was leaving, he said to me, 'I'm afraid I would not have enough to pay you. Would it be alright if you sent me the bill?' I said 'Of course,' being relieved that I did not have to bring up such an embarrassing subject. I saw him down the stairs and just as he got to the door, he said, 'Sure maybe I do have enough to pay you. What's your fee?' I blurted out 'Three guineas', being fearful that he would collapse with dismay and shock. 'Ah, sure doctor, I have that and ten times over,' and with that he took out a large bundle of notes and hands me three little green backs. I could detect that his opinion of me as an eminent Dublin specialist plummeted on the spot!

There was a tradition in those early years of giving your first fee to your mother. I might have done so if my financial circumstances were less precarious, and if the rumpled and dirty old red ten shilling note which I earned during my first week in general practice was more presentable.

In my second week in the village I earned five pounds, although to say that I 'earned' it is an exaggeration. It was customary in Ireland at that time for the doctor attending a confinement to receive a five pound note from the mother after the delivery was completed, whether she was a dispensary patient or not. I got an urgent call to attend a woman in a farmhouse away from the village. When I arrived on my bicycle, I found that the woman had had a miscarriage and that the handywoman present had supervised the entire event, so that the patient was comfortable and well settled down by the time I arrived. I went through the motions of feeling her pulse, pronounced her well, complimented the midwife on the successful if unfortunate outcome, and was about to leave the bedside when the patient took a five pound note out from under the pillow and handed it to me. While I was careful enough to take the money, I felt somewhat embarrassed accepting such a munificent fee when the midwife had done the work, and no doubt was paid a pittance for her trouble. I was to learn later that many of the fees received by doctors are at least partly earned by their nursing colleagues.

By the beginning of my third week the word had got around that there was a new doctor from London in the village. I collected twenty-five pounds in fees during this last week, a quite respectable sum at that time. In my third week I also acquired a chauffeuse with a brand-new Land Rover. My driver came down from Thurles every morning to take me on my calls. She was a Dwan from Thurles whose father owned a mineral water factory. Before Miss Dwan arrived on the scene, I had done my calls outside the village on the schoolmaster's bicycle. I felt a new sense of dignity and importance after her arrival, and these feelings must have been conveyed to my patients, because I found myself almost invariably invited to take a glass of wine after each domiciliary visit. The wine was by tradition Sandeman's port. It was probably the equivalent of the 'Priest's Bottle', invariably a drop of Irish whiskey, which was a feature in many country homes in Ireland. Port must have been considered more appropriate for a lesser mortal such as the doctor! When I was leaving the village on my way back to London, I was satisfied that a useful living could be made there in general practice, although whether success depended on having an affluent and comely maiden from Thurles as a chauffeuse is a moot point.

The little hotel is still extant, I believe. I was last there during the general election campaign of 1957, when a crowd of us used to go down to Tipperary every weekend to canvass for my father when he was president of Fine Gael. It was to be his last election, so that a great cohort of Dublin people who were friendly with the family took part in the exercise, some of whom were not even supporters of his party. I am not sure that we did him any favour by participating in the campaign, although he was successful in being elected. I know that the locals were rather bemused by the arrival of this large body of young, middle-class professional types, who one householder contemptuously called 'college boys'. I arrived at this man's doorway with another medical colleague, Donal O'Sullivan. I had a colourful bow tie, a yellow tweed waistcoat designed and made by my sister couturier, Neillí, and a pair of immaculately creased flannels. When he opened the door, he stared at the two of us for a moment. After this unnatural pause, he turned and shouted to his wife somewhere at the back of the house, 'Mary, will ye come up and have a look at the college boys!'

There were a number of other bizarre confrontations between the city slickers and the country people which cannot have helped in the cause we were serving, and which were reminders of the sharp social and cultural divide between the urban and rural populations in those times.

We used to gather in my little hotel on the Sunday evenings after the weekend campaign was completed. We had a supper of sandwiches and Guinness on our first Sunday night there. It was a very wet stormy night and, because the village was off the beaten track, enquiries were made about the best way to the main Cork–Dublin road. We had a cavalcade of five or six cars. I explained that I had done a locum there in 1949 and assured them that I knew the country intimately. I would lead the way to the main road by the safest and shortest route.

We set out at about midnight. It was frightfully wet and stormy. I drove for some eight or ten miles, and after a while I began to feel a little uncertain of my bearings, particularly as driving conditions were so very bad. However, eventually we arrived at the outskirts of a village. It had a vaguely familiar look about it, but it was not until I arrived at the main street that I realised that we were back where we had started! At first I thought in my panic that I should drive through without comment, hoping that my mistake might remain undetected in the storm, but on second thoughts I was sensible enough to realise that such a strategy would only add to my troubles and embarrassment. This, more than any other event in my life, was to tarnish my reputation as a navigator with family and friends for years to come. Subsequently, if I ever expressed a strong opinion about any subject in their presence, I would be reminded of my intimate knowledge of the topography of County Tipperary.

My host and hostess were a delightful and hospitable pair. Like the country people I knew during my childhood holidays in Kerry and later in County Wexford, they and the villagers were the salt of the earth: honest, hardworking, uncomplaining, full of humour and humanity, generous, and entirely non-acquisitive. A Kerryman by the name of O'Shea was resident in the hotel and was the local schoolteacher. O'Shea was a mine of information about the county and about the social background and people of the village. He was entirely uninhibited in his comments about the local scene, and had, thanks to his many years as a national school teacher there, an intimate insight into the circumstances and customs of the people.

On the road to the west there had been about a dozen cottages, some of which, although occupied until recently, were semi-derelict or in almost total ruin. On the other side of the village to the east there were six modern two-storey houses. Apparently the occupants of the worst of the cottages had been moved to the new houses which had been built by the local authority at the beginning of the war. Perhaps because these families were the most irresponsible and improvident, and therefore the least house-proud, by 1949 the new houses were in a sad, dilapidated state, with the gardens run wild and full of rubbish, the boundaries broken and a general air of neglect and untidiness. According to O'Shea, the baths were used for storage and there was hardly one stick of decent furniture in any of the houses. There were many unkempt children to be seen and, according to the teacher, incest and the sexual abuse of children was rife, a subject which has recently received much publicity. He stated that this was common knowledge in and around the village. In answer to my question why nothing was being done to remedy this state of affairs, he replied, 'The guards are aware of the situation but cannot do anything. The local parish priest does not wish to bring any bad publicity on the village, and has vetoed any action on the matter.'

It is a reminder that aberrant sexual behaviour was a common enough feature of Irish society – it is now simply more openly discussed and the awareness of it is greater. The situation in this village had all the ingredients to encourage family sex abuse and incest. Most of the women in these families were worn out with multiple pregnancies, back-breaking work, drudgery, and indifferent and possibly violent and sexually frustrated husbands. Uneducated and poverty-stricken, they had nobody to turn to for solace or relief, except whatever comfort they might have got from their religion and the confessional. The reluctance of our society in the past to face the realities of sex, as manifested by our lack of openness about the subject, by our neglect of sex education, and by our cultural adherence to the Catholic Church's concepts of sex as the occasion of sin except when performed strictly for procreation, are also important and inescapable factors in encouraging sex abuse and incest. And I believe that we can only make the situation worse if, instead of facing the basic social and cultural causes of this multifarious problem in our society, we attempt to eliminate or curb these abuses with legislation, by the imposition of penalties, by starting a witch hunt, and by attempting to solve moral and personal behaviour by the rule of law. Legislation may assuage our conscience and may take the pressure off of our legislators, just as the abortion amendment did some years ago. It will not, however, solve the underlying problem: it will simply drive it further underground and out of reach. It seems to me that better education, a greater openness about sex and its basic importance for each one of us in a society which should value love in all human relations, the easy availability of birth control and a real commitment to raising the standard of living for every citizen along with greater equality and sharing of wealth, may succeed where legislation is bound to fail.

Despite these exceptional circumstances, the villagers had the humanity, generosity, simplicity and security of a stable peasant culture. There was plenty of sin, no doubt, but very little crime. Because their expectations were minimal, they were philosophical about the misfortunes of life and it never occurred to them to seek financial compensation for them, even when mishaps were caused by the negligence of others.

The countryside was also very different then. There were none of the neatly clipped hedges, the loss of the hedgerow tree, the modern bungalow with its comforts and its manicured garden, or the air of prosperity which is evident in the countryside today. The massive untrimmed hedges at the time made it difficult to see the surrounding country, and gave Ireland the aspect which the French tourist finds intriguing and *sauvage*. The poor farmhouses and cottages, and the cabins of the destitute, have all but disappeared, as have the manure heaps which were not uncommonly found in front of them.

Much has changed for the better for the Irish, at least in the material sense if not in terms of human happiness. I have doubts about changes in our moral and spiritual values which appear to have accompanied our material advancement; and I worry about the threat to our grandchildren and future generations as we sin against nature and our beautiful planet.

4

RETURN TO DUBLIN

I returned to St Vincent's Hospital in September 1950 at the invitation of Professor James A. Meenan, Professor of Medicine at St Vincent's and UCD. I went back with a certain kudos – with my membership of the Royal College of Physicians in London and as the first graduate to return to St Vincent's with an extended period of specialist training abroad. My remit was to carry out a thorough examination of the Outpatients' Department of the hospital (the OPD), and to make recommendations about creating a more modern service based on an appointments system and on referral of patients by outside doctors. The task presented to me seemed a reasonable one but its fulfilment was far from easy. The consultants in the OPD were aware of the need to bring the service into line with modern consultant practice.

St Vincent's was a small hospital of about 140 public and about 80 private beds, housed in a few old Georgian buildings, with a large modern nurses' residence at the rear and various annexes and corridors and cubby holes, all obviously added piecemeal and according to immediate exigencies. The inpatient work and the teaching sessions, which earned the consultants the students' fees, were entirely in the hands of the three or four senior physicians and senior surgeons. My teaching was conducted in my outpatient clinic and became an important part of my work, but it was not official, at least in terms of payment or formal recognition by the university.

I drew up a plan which included an appointments and referral system, but whatever progress was made was slow and continued for many years to be jeopardised by the charitable tradition that the hospital dispensary was an open house to the poor of the city, where medical attention and medicines were provided free for all comers. Progress depended largely on new arrivals to the staff who had undergone specialist training abroad. Progress also owed much to a gradual improvement in the social conditions of the Dublin population after the war, to a more sophisticated and demanding clientele, and also by improved general practitioner services in the city.

My most abiding memories of the dispensary in St Vincent's in the forties and fifties were the large motley crowds, the poverty and destitution of the people, the many patients with visible physical disabilities and deformities, and the widespread lack of hygiene. A pervading and sickly body odour was the rule, halitosis was common even among the better educated, and it was evident that many people at that time rarely washed themselves. I can recall examining the legs and feet of patients with serious circulatory disorders; it was necessary in some patients to examine their legs for circulatory changes. I saw foul-smelling feet which must never have been washed, where the toes adhered together by the filth of ages, and where the socks and the remains of other items of clothing were rotting on limbs and body. I saw the chain smokers with charred fingers and the acrid stale smell of tobacco who coughed so violently that they would vomit as a result of their exertions.

One such man complained of violent productive coughing and vomiting every morning. It took me some time to convince him that it was the result of his smoking and not an unrelated bronchial condition. I told him that he would have to stop smoking and I asked him to return in one month so that I could assess progress. He returned as requested, and confessed that he had not stopped but he claimed to have reduced from sixty to forty cigarettes a day. He seemed greatly relieved that, while he was still coughing up copious quantities of sputum, he had stopped vomiting and his breathing had improved!

I was familiar with the work and the aspirations of the Order of the

Irish Sisters of Charity before I entered St Vincent's as a student – I had an aunt in the order – but I came into intimate contact with the sisters when I became a student there, and later a resident doctor and consultant. The Irish Sisters of Charity made a huge contribution to the care of the poor and the sick in Ireland, particularly during the nineteenth and first half of the twentieth centuries. Long before the government or local authorities provided anything but the bare essential medical services through the dispensary system and custodial care in the houses of industry and lunatic asylums, the sisters were providing for the sick poor, the deaf, the blind, the epileptic, the crippled and the mentally handicapped in their many institutions around the country. Like many other Catholic orders, their contribution to the social and educational services will never be fully appreciated, but should never be forgotten. It is irritating today to hear criticism of the charitable orders for circumstances which existed in the past and which are now judged unacceptable in the context of changing modern times.

In my long experience at St Vincent's, I had nothing but admiration and respect for the sisters' dedication to their calling, for their concern for and care of others, and for their constant good humour, optimism and humanity. I personally received much consideration and understanding from them, although I am only one of the many who have experienced their kindness and support. When I left my wife and children in July 1974, much to everybody's surprise, and took three months' sabbatical in Europe accompanied by my French Algerian friend, I expected short shrift from the hospital authorities on my return. Instead, my rehabilitation was assured by the obvious concern of the sisters, who spared no effort to see that I returned fully to the professional and social life of the hospital. In the more liberal circumstances of the new century in Ireland, my aberrant behaviour in 1974 may not seem so unusual; but in the Catholic professional world in which I lived at that time, it was then as exceptional as it was surprising.

I was appointed to the junior staff as a cardiologist on my return in 1950. Relations among the consultants were always excellent during my time, although as junior colleagues we lacked some of the advantages enjoyed by our seniors, such as membership of the medical board and access to teaching fees from the university. Apart from Donagh

O'Donovan, the newly appointed university Professor of Medicine at the time of my arrival, none of my predecessors in St Vincent's had gone through a period of prolonged training abroad.

At the time of my appointment in 1950, there were large numbers of patients with heart valve problems, mostly caused by rheumatic fever, which occupied my attention. Rheumatic fever had by then become much less common because of the introduction of penicillin about five years earlier, but its long-term complications of heart valve damage were still widely seen. Rheumatic heart disease was particularly common amongst the poor, and my busy outpatients' departments in St Vincent's and the Coombe maternity hospital (which I also attended), were initially dominated by patients with these valve problems. By the time I returned to Ireland, most of the structural and functional disturbances of the heart could be diagnosed by trained cardiologists using clinical means with the aid of eyes, ears and hands, and the electrocardiogram and x-rays, but this new knowledge was slow to permeate the profession at large. It was at this time too that the nature of coronary disease and its accurate diagnosis was first established. Very severe and progressive high blood pressure, also caused by damage to the kidneys by rheumatic fever, became a rarity by the end of the 1950s. The more benign form of high blood pressure unrelated to kidney damage remained common but could usually be controlled by appropriate lifestyle changes and by various drugs.

While in London, and later in Dublin, I had a special interest in smoking as a cause of diseases of the leg arteries, a condition called peripheral vascular disease, or PVD. This common disease at the time was a major cause of severe pain when walking, called intermittent elucidation, and in advanced cases could lead to gangrene and even amputation. Various operations were devised to treat the condition but none proved to be of any value. I noticed a tremendous improvement in those who could be induced to stop smoking and to adopt graduated walking; so much so that their symptoms always showed improvement, often dramatic, or led to complete resolution of symptoms. The arterial disease in the legs of these patients was the same as the arterial disease in the heart in coronary heart disease and it was knowledge of this that first inspired me to identify the important role of cigarette smoking in coronary patients. At a later date, I was to describe the success of this conservative treatment of leg vessel disease at a symposium in Dublin the report of which was subsequently published in the *Irish Journal of Medical Science* in 1964.

Despite my involvement in treating rheumatic valve disease and other clinical and teaching activities, I had virtually no access to beds and lacked the facilities to build my own department. There were no existing facilities for more advanced heart investigation. I was also responsible for general medical care, an aspect of my work which I enjoyed very much but one which was to end when I was eventually provided with my own cardiac unit of sixteen beds ten years later in 1961, at the height of the coronary epidemic.

The electrocardiography (ECG) service was controlled by my senior colleague, Dr Patsy O'Farrell, my mentor and immediate senior. He was a general physician but he had an interest in cardiology without having any special training. Nevertheless, he was influential in advancing the specialty by setting up the Irish Cardiac Society after my arrival, with himself as president and me as secretary. He developed the ECG service in the hospital which marked considerable progress at the time. A tiny little cubby hole at the end of the main corridor of the old St Vincent's was his darkroom. Like all the hospital staff in my early years, the morning was spent in the hospital and the afternoons in private consulting rooms in Fitzwilliam Square and its environs; ward rounds were brief and conducted in a hurried manner. O'Farrell appeared to spend most of the morning in his darkroom and then proceeded to the X-ray department where he smoked a few cigarettes and grunted a few words with his X-ray colleagues before leaving for lunch at home.

He was well disposed towards me in a shy and offhand type of way. While widely different in personality, we had a good relationship and I had affection for him which he probably appreciated despite his very impersonal exterior. He had virtually no private practice and appeared to live on the three guinea fees he charged for ECGs, and on his teaching fees. He eventually retired to London in 1960, rather abruptly and to everyone's surprise, and left the field of cardiology and its advancement open for me. He continued to serve the Sisters of Charity in their hospice work in London.

Patsy O'Farrell had been the Irish representative on the Medical Defence Council and president of the joint IMA and BMA before his retirement, and was well known in medico-political circles. He surprised me at the time of his retirement by proposing me, rather than one of my senior colleagues, as the Irish representative on the Medical Defence Council, but his decision must have been vetoed at some higher level. I heard some months later that my senior colleague, Oliver FitzGerald, had been appointed to this fairly prestigious position. O'Farrell also encouraged me to take part in medical politics by becoming active in the Irish Medical Association; he hoped that I would some day become president of the Association, which I did in 1970. As chairman of the IMA and as president of the Royal College of Physicians of Ireland, he had the shortest fuse imaginable during meetings. As discussion on a subject continued, he would show his impatience by starting to tap his right foot and as his impatience mounted the tapping became more rapid, more vigorous and more audible until he finally insisted on foreclosing the discussion.

The hospital south of the city in Cabinteely had been established by two women paediatricians who were concerned about the number of children with rheumatic and congenital heart disease. Rheumatic heart disease was the result of active rheumatic fever, which tended to present in young children in a low grade and prolonged fashion, and which at times gave rise to some difficulties in establishing the presence or absence of disease.

The two doctors in charge invited me to visit their sanatorium in Cabinteely where I spent a morning examining about forty young patients. I found the exercise to be both revealing and embarrassing. More than half the patients I examined had innocent murmurs. (Murmurs are sounds caused by blood flow turbulence in the heart or blood vessels, which may be caused by structural abnormalities in the heart and vessels or may be entirely innocent, normal disturbances in blood flow. I learned to distinguish innocent from organic heart murmurs during my training and in children such innocent murmurs are particularly common.) These children had no evidence of a convincing history to support the diagnosis of rheumatic fever. Symptoms of joint pains were not convincing and, for want of a better word, we used the term 'growing pains' to explain any non-specific complaint of pain which might have been elicited. With the modern echocardiogram, it is easy to distinguish the significance of any murmur which may be found, so that the modern cardiologist is less dependent on his stethoscope and I fear may be losing some clinical skills.

I cannot recall exactly how I expressed my views to the two doctors concerned, but I expect that I was reasonably diplomatic in saying that at least some of the murmurs were of no significance, particularly if the relevant blood tests were normal. I do not know if my visit served any useful purpose as I received no further invitations to visit the clinic, but in the early 1950s there was widespread misdiagnosis of heart murmurs and of other perceived heart conditions which led to unnecessary lifestyle restrictions.

I saw a patient for a routine check-up at the Charlemont Clinic shortly before I retired from there. He was aged fifty-three and was perfectly healthy. His parents informed him that at the age of five I had seen him because of a murmur and was able to reassure his parents that the murmur was functional and of no significance. My patient informed me that, prior to seeing me when he was a child, his parents had been advised by several doctors that he should be prevented from taking part in normal childhood activities, and, in one case, the doctor advised the parents to keep him 'in cotton wool' in case the heart condition might be aggravated by exercise. This type of prohibition of exercise was all too common in these early days.

After my arrival at St Vincent's, my outpatient clinic was soon invaded by hordes of students wishing to learn the physical signs of valve disease and other cardiac disorders. They arrived after the official teaching sessions which were held each weekday morning from 9 to 11. It was necessary to confine the invasion to final-year students, all of whom were anxious to face the rigours of the final examination and to be familiar with the newly described signs of heart disease. It was still the time when exact diagnosis depended on careful history-taking, and on the evidence provided by the eyes, ears and hands. These were the halcyon days of bedside clinical medicine.

My students and residents will recall the intense interest we had in identifying murmurs and other audible, visible and palpable signs which allowed us to make confident diagnoses of structural changes in the heart muscle or valves. Accuracy in clinical diagnosis was not established until after the war when some cardiologists, in Britain and America in particular, through careful clinical observation and with the assistance X-ray and of catheter findings introduced into the heart chambers through a blood vessel, were successful in the course of a few years in giving clinical diagnosis a firm, rational basis. The catheter was a thin tube by which pressures could be measured and dye could be introduced to identify structural changes by X-ray. It was also only after the war that a clear appreciation of the pathology and the different forms of coronary heart disease emerged in the same medical and research centres.

HEART VALVE SURGERY AND RESEARCH

When I returned to Ireland I joined Bob O'Connell in establishing a cardiac surgery service at St Vincent's Hospital. Prior to my arrival, Bob and his colleague, Paddy Fitzgerald, had done a few operations on the main arteries of the chest which had been recently performed successfully abroad. Our new service was based on operating on the patients who had a rheumatic valve disease called mitral stenosis. This operation had recently been developed in the United States.

Bob O'Connell was one of those larger than life surgeons, brimming with confidence. His conversation and speeches were replete with stories and jokes. He was a political animal and was active in the Irish Medical Association. As a leading member of the Association, his was the influence which scuppered Noel Browne's Mother and Health Child Scheme and which contributed to the demise of the first Inter-party Government.

Our new surgical service was limited to mitral valve surgery, and to repairing some major blood vessel anomalies in the chest. We were to wait another two decades or more before the development of the pump oxygenator allowed a greatly increased scope of treatment through open heart surgery. On my return, we had started doing an operation to relieve the obstructed mitral valve, which proved to be reasonably successful although it was a relatively crude form of surgery compared to subsequent more elegant and more efficient forms of valve replacement. Mitral stenosis was invariably caused by rheumatic fever; the result of infection by the haemolytic streptococcus. Rheumatic fever occurred mostly in children and young people. Inflammation of the mitral valve and, less commonly, the aortic valve, was a common sequel during its active inflammatory stages and was frequently followed by healing of the valve leaflets and constriction of the valve. The constricted valve was amenable to widening by a finger or knife inserted through the upper chamber of the heart. By simple clinical examination the trained cardiologist could identify the severity of the constriction, exclude significant leakage, and so decide on the cases which were suitable for operation.

The streptococcus which caused rheumatic fever was widespread, particularly among the poor because of overcrowding, poor nutrition and their appalling housing conditions. But by the time I returned to Dublin rheumatic fever was in rapid decline due to the high sensitivity of the streptococcus to antibiotics, and particularly to penicillin. For some reason this particular valve lesion was more common in women than in men, hence it was particularly common among the poor women to whom I attended in the Coombe Lying-in Hospital during their pregnancies.

In the early 1960s, there was intense interest in the development of open-heart surgery. Earlier, and apart from the relatively crude mitral operation, it was impossible to operate on the heart valves or coronary vessels because of the need to suspend the circulation. Brain damage and death is inevitable if the heart stops for three minutes or more at the normal body temperature of 37 degrees. In the late 1960s, we started research work on open-heart surgery at St Vincent's Hospital at a time when it was also proceeding in the Mater Hospital in Dublin and in other countries. Two approaches were feasible and both were being actively researched. One was the heart/lung machine based on a pump to take over from the heart and an oxygenator to add oxygen to the blood and extract carbon dioxide. This method was pioneered by the Hammersmith Hospital in London and was adopted by the Mater in Dublin.

The other approach was profound hypothermia. Here, the patient's temperature was lowered to about 25 degrees. At this temperature, the brain can survive without circulation and without life-giving oxygen for an hour or two. The heart stops beating at about 31 degrees, which allows direct access to the inert heart, its valves and arteries. Profound hypothermia was developed by Charles Drew and his colleagues at the Westminster Hospital in London and was the approach adopted by us at St Vincent's Hospital. It was to the Westminster Hospital that our team of two surgeons, an anaesthetist, a technician and myself went to familiarise ourselves with the technique and to start our own research programme at home.

There was an old two-storey house at the back of St Vincent's Hospital with its rear to the Loreto School. It had been a piggery which was maintained discretely by the nuns but which was eventually closed in the late fifties because of more stringent urban hygiene laws introduced by the Corporation. We gained access to this building as an animal research lab. For a variety of reasons we decided that the pig was the most suitable animal for experimentation. Or perhaps it would be more accurate to say that it was the least unsuitable. We completed about twenty experiments in all, achieving a certain measure of success in cooling the pig, opening the chest, handling the heart, stitching up and returning the animal to a normal temperature. No pig survived and only a few returned to a transient living state. The pig's arteries were small and friable and hence difficult to handle. The heart too was smaller and less robust than the human heart but the poor quality of the arteries made it difficult to manipulate the vessels and to introduce the large needles, or 'trocars', necessary to provide blood and the cooling fluids.

My function, apart from that of being a spectator, was to provide the pig and the six pints of porcine blood to replace blood loss. Through the good offices of James O'Mara of Donnelly's and Sons in Cork Street, we were regularly provided with a live pig and five to six pints of pig's blood. I visited the factory to collect the pig and the blood in the late morning before each experiment commenced. I was accompanied on each occasion by an enthusiastic and willing young resident house physician, Michael Murphy. We arrived in my old Rover car to where the pigs were housed in a concrete compound in the factory.

The pigs in the factory were disposed of by severing the carotid arteries in the neck with an efficient machete. Michael or myself advanced in white surgical coats and hats, stood beneath the pig at the vital moment when a torrent of blood doused the platform. We had a large basin which we held at the correct spot and, after a few pigs were disposed of, we had sufficient blood to fill five or six pint bottles. The noise was infernal. It was created by the pigs in the compound, the pig on its way to eternity, the grating noise of the equipment and the other extraneous sounds of a busy factory.

As we left with the cache of blood, we packed a live pig into a strong hessian bag, put the sack into the boot of my car and returned to the hospital and our animal laboratory.

I always stopped the car at the corner of the L-shaped lane at the back of the hospital close to the nuns' old piggery. On one occasion, when we opened the boot the pig jumped out and left both of us standing. The animal had managed to escape from the bag while in transit; he raced, squealing, up the lane and arrived at top speed at O'Reilly's pharmacy in Leeson Street with the two of us in our bloodstained white coats chasing after him. He took a left turn – it was not a one-way street at the time – and we followed him up as far as Hatch Street, where we lost him. It wasn't until the pig had disappeared up towards Leeson Street Bridge, and our exertions came to an end, that we became conscious of the gaping spectators who must have been astonished by the bizarre nature of the hectic and bloody scene. We never solved the mystery of the pig's ultimate destination and we were lucky to scurry back to the hospital without being locked up.

Charles Drew (later Sir Charles), who had pioneered the technique at the Westminster Hospital in London, came over to supervise and assist and to launch us on our learning curve. The first human subject had an abnormal opening between the two main chambers of the heart. He was first put to sleep and was then cooled by running cooling fluid through a vein and immersing him in an ice-cold bath. The internal body temperature was continually monitored. At about 31 degrees centigrade the heart developed ventricular fibrillation, an electrical disturbance which prevents the heart from beating regularly and efficiently and which stops the circulation to the body. By this time the brain is reasonably well protected from lack of oxygen. The temperature is brought down further in the bath to about 25 degrees. When the operation is completed and the chest closed, the patient is reheated externally and by warmed blood. At about 31 to 32 degrees, the heart may start to beat spontaneously or may be restarted by an electric shock administered by a defibrillator.

The first patient's operation was completed successfully and he survived. We carried out about twenty operations in all with mixed results. The method proved cumbersome, some of the patients had advanced conditions and our small hospital, with poor facilities for such specialised work, was unsuitable. At the same time the heart/lung machine was proving more successful and more practical at the Hammersmith in London and it was clear that the Mater Hospital, led by Professor Eóin O'Malley, had made the right decision. To the best of my knowledge, the technique of profound hypothermia as an adjunct to open heart surgery is not routinely used except in rare conditions to assist the heart/lung machine.

Despite all the work by O'Connell and his younger surgical colleagues, we supported the resolution proposed at a meeting of the Irish Cardiac Society that the Mater should become the national cardiac surgery centre. A considerable degree of chauvinism prevailed in some of our hospitals at the time, particularly between St Vincent's and the Mater. Our decision to terminate the open-heart surgery service at St Vincent's Hospital was at first greeted with dismay by our senior colleagues. We had chosen the loser in terms of our approach to open-heart surgery and we agreed with our colleagues in the Irish Cardiac Society that Ireland should be served by one properly organised and sufficiently funded heart surgery centre. The Mater was chosen because of its heart/lung approach and its greater size and access to patients. To achieve optimum results in heart surgery and in other complex areas of surgery, one must have an adequate number of patients to train and ensure the expertise of the surgeon and the surgical team. At that time in Ireland this condition could only be fulfilled by one centre.

Our decision proved a godsend to coronary and surgery patients because of our own major subsequent contributions to coronary heart disease prevention and research, and to the success of the first large coronary care unit which was set up at St Vincent's in 1966. The decision also contributed to the Mater's great success as Ireland's national heart surgical centre.

THE COOMBE LYING-IN HOSPITAL

Shortly after my return to Ireland I was approached by Dr Kevin Feeney, who was then Master of the Coombe Lying-in Hospital, to join his staff and to look after the many women of child-bearing age who were suffering from rheumatic heart disease, and who, because of their heart condition, were a major source of morbidity and mortality in the maternity service. The appointment of non-obstetricians in the maternity service at the time was only commencing. Previously the Coombe would call on a surgeon or physician from St Vincent's in the event of an emergency.

I established a weekly clinic there where all the heart and other medical patients were seen by me. Rheumatic heart disease was still a particular scourge among the poorer classes in Ireland and particularly in women. I saw patients with rheumatic heart disease of varying severity and at various stages of pregnancy. The social conditions of many of them were poor, particularly in terms of malnutrition, iron deficiency anaemia and chronic respiratory infections. These were major complicating factors in the heart patients and so often helped to precipitate heart failure. There is little doubt that when the patients received optimum medical treatment, combined later with much improved social circumstances, their prognoses were greatly improved, even without surgery. It was impossible not to have a regard and an admiration for these women who, despite their poverty, multiparity and perceived hardship, maintained such good humour and acceptance of their lot based on a sense of community and their commitment to the Catholic faith.

With Bob O'Connell, and later Gussy Mehigan, we relieved a number of patients with obstructed valves by operation during their pregnancy. In other cases, where the operation was not feasible, we dealt with patients as best we could by appropriate rest, by using the very limited drugs which were available to us at the time, and by treating anaemia or other aggravating factors. In fact, we had relatively few deaths from heart disease during these early years, although it remained the most prevalent medical cause of obstetrical death in Ireland until the 1970s. By the end of the 1970s or the early 1980s, cases of rheumatic heart disease in pregnancy became a rarity and my duties at the Coombe Lying-in hospital were greatly alleviated. Of the 150 patients who were subjected to surgery under my care in my two hospitals, the most dramatic case was the patient who had gone into rapid heart failure while in labour and had emergency surgery in the delivery room. Both mother and child survived.

I continued to do a weekly clinic in the Coombe up to the time of my retirement in 1988. I was joined by my friend and colleague Professor William O'Dwyer in the late 1970s. He was a kidney specialist who was the first in Ireland to introduce dialysis for kidney failure. He was Professor of Medicine in the Charitable Infirmary, Jervis Street and the

Royal College of Surgeons. My family was fortunate that he taught my two sons, David and Hugh, the important rudiments of medicine and they ultimately qualified in medicine under his wing. Billy was appointed to the Coombe Hospital at my suggestion because of his interest in high blood pressure and kidney disease, conditions which replaced heart disease as the major medical problems to be encountered in pregnancy. I also had a lifetime interest in high blood pressure and later published our research results of high blood pressure in pregnancy, particularly in the case of its management by drugs. I was glad to have O'Dwyer as a colleague; it allowed me to share with him the responsibility of doing the clinical work and of dealing with emergency situations.

By the 1980s the size of my clinic at the Coombe had been greatly reduced and my most important duty was to be available for medical emergencies. However, I did have one rather unusual function as a physician in these later years. Shortly after the contraceptive pill was introduced, I believe in the early 1970s, it was generally accepted and prescribed by the obstetricians in the hospital. However, these obstetricians were a conservative lot and were greatly dominated by the influence of the Catholic Church in terms of medical matters, and shortly afterwards they refused to prescribe the pill as part of family planning. No group of patients needed this effective method of family planning more than the numerous multiparous, economically deprived and disadvantaged patients who made up a large proportion of those attending the hospital. However, with a very conservative Catholic archbishop as the chairman of the hospital board, my obstetrical colleagues were obviously influenced by his disapproval of this 'sinful' form of family planning. I am afraid the Catholic Church must share the blame, along with Muslims and other fundamentalist religious groups, for the disastrous increase in the world human population, which is part of the forthcoming crisis facing the human race and the root cause of the depletion of the planet's natural resources.

I had no compunctions about prescribing the pill and one of my functions was prescribing it for patients who came to me specifically for this purpose. I cannot recall that my aberrant intervention in this matter caused any concern to my obstetrical colleagues. They never spoke to me about the matter, nor did the master ever intervene despite his and his colleagues' reluctance to prescribe the pill. Referring to the very conservative approach of the obstetricians to such matters as family planning and to their strict adherence to the teaching of the Church, it may be relevant to point out that the Coombe owed its origin entirely to secular influences, and largely to Arthur Guinness and Co. On two occasions during the nineteenth century, the hospital was threatened with closure because of lack of money. On each occasion it was rescued by the munificence of the firm of Arthur Guinness, which of course had extensive properties in and close to the Coombe area. The old hospital was situated in the Coombe, close to the Liberties. It was moved to a new site in Rialto beside the Grand Canal around 1970. The wards and theatres in the old Coombe had secular names; the wards in the new Coombe were called after various saints, some of whom were little known to me, such as Saint Monica, and some of whom have already been removed from the calendar of saints by the liberal Pope John XXIII.

I recall writing to the Medical Board commenting on the hospital's new policy of paying tribute to the Roman Catholic saints in this way. I expressed regret that no ward or other section of the hospital was named to pay tribute to the important part the Guinness family had played in maintaining the hospital, particularly at the times it was threatened with closure, not to mention the fact that the brewery supplied the hospital free of charge with a daily supply of stout for all the patients. This tradition continued during my time on the staff until the arrangement ceased, perhaps after the transfer of the hospital to the Rialto site. I do not think that I got a reply to my letter, nor did the hospital respond to my suggestion.

I have a liberal view about abortion up to the twelfth week of pregnancy, mainly because I am more concerned about the serious effect the population explosion is likely to have on nature and on the future of the human race. Humanity is in serious denial about the issue and the inevitable disaster facing this and future generations. It is a concern which greatly exceeds my reservations about the moral issues of abortion. We may have to change our moral norms. Nevertheless I cannot recall any case during my professional work at the Coombe Lying-in Hospital where I could say confidently that an abortion would have been necessary for the survival of the mother. It is for this reason that I have great doubts about the opinion of many Irish people and of our Supreme Court judges that abortion should be prohibited except in cases where the mother's life might be endangered by the pregnancy. If this proposition is accepted no doubt many women will have their pregnancies terminated because of a professional opinion that the pregnancy represents a threat to their health or interferes with some life-giving medical intervention which in itself causes interruption of pregnancy.

Society should decide one way or another, either to prohibit abortion under all circumstance or to allow it to be performed only in the early stages of pregnancy and at the request of the mother. It is believed that there are currently about seven thousand elective abortions every year among Irish women visiting the UK, an abortion rate of 0.6 percent of the entire child-bearing female population. If we apply these figures to the world population of close seven billion, I would estimate that there are 12 million abortions worldwide every year, which is a relatively small fraction of the estimated 80 million annual increase in the world population. My guess is that this is a very conservative estimate and that the annual global abortion rate may be substantially greater than the rate for Ireland where all the abortions are performed abroad.

In the late 1960s I initiated a research programme at the Coombe on various aspects of maternal smoking and reproductive health. I was subsequently joined in this research by Dr John Murphy, who later joined the consultant staff of the National Maternity Hospital in Holles Street. We published seven papers in the national and international medical press confirming a higher prevalence of miscarriage and stillbirth in the smoking women and a substantially lower birth weight among the smoking women who had reached full term. The reduced birth weight of the infants made them more prone to neo-natal problems.

OTHER ACTIVITIES DURING THE 1950S AND 1960S

My first ten years on the staff of St Vincent's Hospital was a relatively quiet time in my professional life although we had made an important contribution to mitral valve surgery. I started publishing papers from my arrival in St Vincent's on a variety of medical subjects; my principle publications being related to the results of our treatment of mitral stenosis. At this time I became interested in the lives of the Dublin physicians of the nineteenth century. There was a period then when the Dublin school of medicine was famous for its contribution to medical science. Some of the physicians in Dublin – Stokes, Corrigan, Cheyne and others – were names well known worldwide for their contributions to the diagnosis and treatment of heart disease. During the 1960s I published seven papers about their contributions, written from the point of view of our modern perspective of heart disease.

Shortly after I had returned to St Vincent's Hospital, I was invited by the then Mother General of the Irish Sisters of Charity to take day-to-day charge of the postulants who were housed in the mother house. My duties included an initial medical examination prior to the entry of each candidate to the order and making a routine visit every week to see anyone deemed to be in need of medical attention. My commitment to care for the young nuns was by way of an invitation but it was quite clear, in the context of the authoritarianism at the time, that a refusal to do so would not be acceptable. In fact, it was clearly intended to be an honour rather than a duty. Emergencies were rare and I cannot say that during the ten or twelve years of my commitment I once saw a case of serious illness. They were a healthy lot and were obviously well cared for by the order during their novitiate.

Mother General undertook to pay me £100 annually for my services, but no payment was forthcoming until three years later when I mentioned to one of the sisters at St Vincent's that the arrangement had never been honoured. A few weeks later, I got a cheque for £100. During the rest of my services, which lasted in all about twelve years, I never received another cheque. By the end of my stint with her precious postulants I was earning enough to accept my role as an honorary one. In the 1950s, authority in the order's institutions was absolute and implacable, a situation which would be perceived today as onerous and dictatorial. But whatever resentment we may have felt towards our masters (and I cannot recall any such resentment) was more than compensated for by the greater sense of security and public order which prevailed then; compared to the personal power and freedom, often without an equal degree of responsibility, which is a feature of our society today.

Also in my early days in St Vincent's, I was invited to act as medical officer to Our Lady's Hospice of the Dying at Harold's Cross. The Hospice, the forerunner of the hospice movement worldwide, was established by the Sisters of Charity in 1888. The Sisters were greatly respected by the population of Ireland for their work in the hospice and elsewhere. Like many other Irish orders, their work and services, their *Caritas Christi*, was carried abroad to many other lands.

Dr John O'Callaghan, a general practitioner working in the city centre, was already installed as a medical officer in the hospice. My arrival on the scene provided him with a well-earned rest every second week. Nowadays, a trained cardiologist would never start his or her consultant career by looking after the chronic sick or the dying, but I had little choice in the 1950s when specialisation was in its infancy, and the boundaries between different medical disciplines were less clearly defined. Indeed, my experience in general practice while in training and my general medical duties at St Vincent's and at the hospice during my early consultant days added a new dimension to my development as a mature and committed physician. It is impossible to work in a hospice without being moved by the devotion of the sisters and nursing staff, the sense of security and the consolations provided to the sick and dying. I attended the hospice daily, except Sunday, every second week. I lived quite near Harold's Cross. I expect that I was paid for my services but, if I am to judge the monetary rewards of service at the time, it must have been a pittance.

The process of dying there was very different from today's circumstances. We did not 'officiously' keep patients alive who were clearly at a semi-terminal or terminal stage. We had neither the complex nor multiple diagnostic modalities at our disposal, nor had we a huge pharmacopoeia or the inclination for patients to survive beyond their natural span. Policy was to keep patients as comfortable and pain-free as possible and to provide them with a sense of security and comfort, and, for some, of spiritual resignation. We were not faced by the current ethical, legal and financial problems which prevail in our major hospitals in dealing with the chronic sick, the dependent invalid and those who are close to or at a terminal stage of disease. Despite recent advances in the management of chronic pain, including the availability of pain clinics and physicians with special skills in this area, I cannot recall that chronic pain was a major problem in patient management. We used the Brompton mixture liberally where appropriate. This soothing medicine contained heroin, cocaine and morphine, and was as well known in these times as Valium is today. We had many patients with advanced or terminal cancer. Cancer of the stomach was common then as were cancers of the breast, colon, skin and prostate. One had an opportunity of learning about the natural history of cancer, for many patients were admitted who had not been subjected to surgery or to anti-cancer drugs which were not then available. It was remarkable that many cancer patients survived after admission for long periods, as long as two or more years, showing little evidence of symptomatic or physical decline until undergoing rapid deterioration before death. I expect that such long-term survivors eventually succumbed when secondary deposits invaded the vital abdominal organs, the brain and the bone marrow.

I mention my experience of cancer patients who were not subjected to the surgical, radiation or other interventions which are widely practised today. It would be foolish to deny that huge advances have been made in the management of cancer, particularly in the early stages, during the last half century. But one might well ask if today's oncologists and surgeons who are dealing with the more advanced stages of cancer have any personal knowledge of the natural history of cancer in the later stages; and whether the benefits of dealing strenuously with the more advanced cases is better, in terms of quality of life, complications and longevity, than adopting a conservative approach aimed at alleviating symptoms, providing the psychological and social support which palliative care nurses and physicians are trained to do, and avoiding unnecessary institutional care and medical interventions.

Apart from cancer, other cases I can vividly recall are severe strokes, patients with advanced rheumatoid arthritis and neurological disorders such as multiple sclerosis and motor neurone disease. The patients with rheumatoid arthritis were a pitiful sight, bedridden with their severe contractures, simulating the foetal position, a picture which is rarely seen nowadays thanks to great advances in drug treatment and to highly effective rehabilitation and physiotherapy programmes.

MY PERSONAL LIFE AT THIS TIME

My early years in Dublin left me with much leisure time. I became interested in bridge and on a few occasions I found myself playing every evening of the week. I also became an active member of my two golf clubs, Milltown and Portmarnock. Despite these many activities, I followed the custom of my colleagues at the hospital by visiting patients twice daily, in the morning and evening. We did not have the backup of competent residents at the time. Because of my limited inpatient responsibilities, mostly acting for senior colleagues, my visits were generally short. On one occasion I had under my care a young man dying from advanced rheumatic heart disease. I had been out in Portmarnock playing golf and stayed too long in the bar afterwards to consider it wise to pay my evening visit to the hospital. It was long before the prohibitions of drink driving. Next morning I learnt that he had died that night and shortly after my arrival in the hospital I was asked to visit the Reverend Mother.

'Dr Mulcahy,' she said on my arrival, 'when you were appointed to this hospital as a heart specialist, you were expected to carry out your duties in a professional and responsible manner. I fear that your absence yesterday evening when your patient was dying was not consistent with these obligations. I have been informed recently that you are becoming an expert golf and bridge player. I am asking you now to decide if you would prefer to become a professional golf and bridge player or would you prefer to remain in this hospital as a physician. I would be obliged if you could make that decision now.'

I left her office feeling humiliated and perhaps somewhat aggrieved. I continued to play bridge and, although I became captain of my home golf club, Milltown, in 1954, I pursued these leisure activities a little more circumspectly. I continued in St Vincent's Hospital, in the Coombe Lying-in Hospital and in our Lady's Hospice.

My entry into private practice, my only source of income, was a slow and gradual process. I shared rooms in Bill Doolin's house at No. 2 Fitzwilliam Square with my colleague, Oliver McCullen, who joined the St Vincent's staff about my time as an ear, nose and throat surgeon. We had my cousin, Maura Mulcahy, as our secretary from the beginning. She had made a miraculous recovery from pulmonary tuberculosis and a recent thoracoplasty. Her father was Paddy Mulcahy, who shortly afterwards became chief of staff of the army, thirty-seven years after his older brother, my father Richard, held the same post during the War of Independence. At Paddy's request, I took her on to assist her rehabilitation after she had spent a few years in a sanatorium. Her father saw it as an act of charity but it was one which paid me rich dividends, for she remained a most loyal and dedicated partner and friend during my thirty-eight years in St Vincent's Hospital. Despite an apparently fragile constitution, she remained in good health during these years. It was not until she retired to look after her aging stepmother, Polly, that I finally recognised how much she had relieved me of the burden of the many everyday problems which would otherwise have created intolerable stresses in my busy professional life.

In my first year in private practice I grossed £240 and in my second £480. There were none of the immediate and handsome rewards which the young cardiologists can expect as soon as they start consultant practice in Ireland today, nor did we receive any remuneration from our hospitals, unlike the handsome salary the present consultants receive. It required seven years to pay off my overdraft of £2,000 which I had accumulated by 1950 at the time of my return to Ireland. Yet, I cannot recall being in any way preoccupied by the subject of money, and I believe that it was not until later years, when I found myself more independent financially, that I developed any sense of acquisitiveness. In my early and impecunious years, I enjoyed the poker and bridge we played for unaffordable stakes in Milltown Golf Club and elsewhere. My interest in gambling gradually waned as I acquired more of this world's goods. I was lucky that the modest beginnings of my career protected me from the temptations of acquiring money for money's sake. When we think of money, we need to remember the words of Jeremy Bentham: 'Without too much, one cannot have enough.' And the Romans reminded us: *crescit amor nummi, quantum ipsa pecunnia crescit* ('the greater the wealth, the greater the love of money').

5

THE HEART DEPARTMENT AT ST VINCENT'S HOSPITAL 1960–1988

Our coronary care unit at St Vincent's Hospital was established in June 1966. It was a quantum leap in the management of coronary heart disease, particularly in its acute stages. It contributed hugely to our understanding of the natural history of the disease; it allowed us to identify the precursors of complications and it provided an effective means of preventing and treating heart rhythm disturbances and heart failure. It also involved the entire medical team in the immediate and long-term management of the coronary patient.

The importance of the coronary care unit is that patients at high risk of sudden death (ventricular fibrillation) and other acute complications can be dealt with immediately by trained staff with access to appropriate equipment. Lives can be saved by immediate cardio-respiratory resuscitation, by electric defibrillation and by reversing the clotting in the affected artery. If the damage to the heart is extensive it may need immediate measures to prevent irreversible heart failure.

The precise diagnosis of the coronary syndromes and their precise nomenclature was not understood by cardiologists until after the Second World War, before I returned from training in London. Diagnosis was greatly facilitated by the advent of the electrocardiogram (ECG), first invented in the early twentieth century in Eindhoven in the Netherlands. However, it only became widely available in hospitals in the late 1940s and early 1950s. Pioneering work on the identification of cardiac irregularities had already taken place in the 1920s and the 1930s, but all these applications were slow to extend to the diagnosis of coronary disease. However, the ECG eventually played a crucial part in clarifying the various coronary syndromes. We were to wait some more years to get the more sophisticated treadmill or bicycle ergometer machines, with which stress testing could be carried out more efficiently. By exercise stress testing we could identify diagnostic changes of coronary disease which might not be present in the ordinary resting ECG.

Stress testing has other applications beyond the diagnosis of heart disease. It can further guide us about prognosis and treatment; it is a useful measure of fitness, which in itself is a valuable guide to health; it provides baseline information about appropriate exercise programmes which may be prescribed; it is also a routine investigation in physiological research and in the more sophisticated sports centres it provides an aid about the potential and the training of elite athletes.

After the Second World War, the importance of careful clinical evaluation was appreciated for the first time as investigations, such as the ECG, radiology and the development of cardiac catheterisation, became available in heart research centres. It was then that improved international communication at a clinical and research level added to our knowledge of heart irregularities, coronary heart disease, congenital heart disease and valve diseases of the heart.

During the 1950s and 1960s, as the incidence of coronary heart disease increased and even as our diagnostic precision improved, treatment of the condition had no rational basis. The cause of the epidemic was unknown and no specific drugs or any other forms of intervention were available. The traditional treatment was based on prolonged rest, on the avoidance of exercise, frequently on discouraging a return to work, and generally on the rationale of resting the heart and on a variety of instructions which bore no relationship whatever to rational management. When we moved to the new site of St Vincent's Hospital in Elm Park in 1971, I was provided with a purpose-built coronary care unit designed and based on my five-year experience of coronary care at St Stephen's Green and by visits to other units in the United Kingdom and the United States. The patients were monitored continuously and could be seen from a common consol where the nurses had a full view of the patients and immediate access to aid and equipment if an emergency were to arise.

There was the problem of providing separate accommodation for men and women because, with the greater number of male admissions and as the unit was almost invariably fully occupied, it was necessary to have a mixed ward. There was no precedent at the time for such an arrangement but, despite the concern of some of my medical and nursing colleagues, this solution was readily agreed to by our secretary manager. It was an innovation but it worked well and without any embarrassment or inconvenience. Indeed, it may have led to a few enduring relationships!

The cardiac department at the time consisted of sixteen beds, two outpatient sessions per week, undergraduate teaching responsibilities, and a department of research including a research doctor and nurse, a secretary, a dietician and a part-time statistician. It included my colleague, Dr Noel Hickey, as a physician and epidemiologist and it was joined later in 1978 for a period of five years by Dr Ian Graham, now professor of cardiology attached to Tallaght Hospital and a now-prominent figure in international cardiovascular epidemiology. Dr Brian Maurer joined as a second clinical cardiologist in 1974 when he became the director of the diagnostic angiology facility and joined me in running the coronary care unit.

It may seem surprising in the strict non-smoking environment of today that our decision in 1971 to prohibit smoking in the cardiac wards was considered revolutionary by the hospital staff. However, it was successful from the beginning and received the full co-operation of staff and patients. I did a ward round every Monday, Wednesday and Friday mornings accompanied by ward sister, a few staff nurses or nurses in training, resident medical staff and perhaps a scattering of students and an occasional visitor. Afterwards I would respond to consultation requests in the other wards of the hospital. Monday was taken up mostly in seeing new patients who had been admitted over the weekend, but the nature of the rounds did not differ from day to day. Wednesday was the most detailed and longest round because of a greater emphasis on teaching on that day. I used to start each day at ten o'clock and finish about midday on Mondays and Fridays, and on Wednesdays I could continue until lunch time or later.

During ward sessions I would seat myself beside each patient, ask for the details of history and examination from the resident responsible for the preliminary investigation, and then examine the patient and often enquire further into the patient's history. Sitting beside the bedside was important because it established an empathy with the patient, particularly as I made a rule of touching the patient at some stage of the process, feeling the pulse or doing a more detailed examination. It also saved me the fatigue of prolonged standing which was the fate of all the others who attended. Apart from an occasional fainting attack, those attending the rounds seemed to tolerate the prolonged upright position without complaint.

In the early 1980s, I was running marathons and I was much fitter than any member of my staff in the hospital. My resting heart rate in bed at that time counted as low as 44. It is now about 56 as I am fit for my age, thanks to my cycling, walking and playing golf. After rounds in the coronary unit, which was on the ground floor, I would visit the other wards to see patients at the request of colleagues. The semi-private ward, St Michael's, was on the fourth floor. I usually had a patient or two there and I would commence my peripatetic consultations by running up the four flights. I was well able to control my breathing when I got to the top and I had a brief moment to recover before the rest of the group arrived, somewhat physically distressed and even a little embarrassed by the performance of somebody who was more than twice their age. It was one of my few attempts of one-upmanship. About the same time I organised a hospital team to run in the Dublin marathon. Several members of the female staff joined in the preliminary training bouts until some enthusiast in the group, no doubt encouraging the girls, said at a meeting that running was good to develop the leg muscles. Few of the females continued to participate after that 'helpful' remark.

We did not do 'cold' rounds then as they do nowadays, when the notes of the patients are discussed in the day room or lecture theatre away from the ward with the entire clinical staff, after the patients are seen by the resident doctor. The patient may or may not be rolled in during the discussion for further evaluation. Ward rounds are now more perfunctory, at least as far as the consultants are concerned, and there appears to be much less teaching at the ward level. The old and long-established apprentice system, first started by the great Irish physicians of the early nineteenth century, where the student was part of the clinical team and followed the consultant during his entire rounds and consultations in the hospital, appears to have been overtaken by the 'cold' rounds, the lecture theatre and the laboratory – a change attributed to the students' more academic education at the undergraduate level and partly induced by the different patterns of illness the consultants are dealing with nowadays.

The type of patient problems that doctors and hospitals are dealing with today are very different from what we dealt with thirty or more years ago. The nature of heart disease has changed since the early days when valve disease and congenital heart disease were rampant and largely diagnosed through bedside examination. Today the relative rarity of these conditions makes it understandable that the bedside examination has less priority but the place of history-taking is as important as it was in the past. The modern public teaching hospital is increasingly concerned with acute problems and is fully equipped to treat all emergency work. There are fewer elective patients admitted, unlike the situation in my earlier years. Many elective patients admitted then can now be dealt with as outpatients. The accident and emergency department is now the heart of our public hospitals and the more leisurely clinical circumstances our nurses and doctors enjoyed in the past have become more frenetic. Our two-tier system of health care, which has been encouraged by our current minister, includes many new private hospitals which cannot deal with many of the acute problems and which are unlikely to play a comprehensive part in dealing with our health problems while adding significantly to health costs.

I first attended 'cold' rounds in Iowa City in 1972 when I spent a week in the local university hospital as visiting professor. During the week I did not once visit the wards until I asked to be shown around the coronary care unit. All contact with the consultant staff was in the lecture theatre or in their offices. Most patients discussed in the theatre were not present, although one lady of ninety-two years with a patent ductus (an abnormal blood vessel in the chest) and heart failure was wheeled in before a decision was made about the advisability of surgery. I cannot remember what decision was arrived at but my conservative attitude to such a problem was certainly jolted by the prospect of submitting the patient to such heroics as surgery although nowadays surgery even in the very elderly is sometimes feasible.

There appears to be less interest in clinical evaluation nowadays among family doctors and much more in arranging investigations and a dependency on their results. Not infrequently, quite elaborate investigations are performed routinely and without adequate initial clinical information. In my practice and that of many of my contemporary colleagues, where the patient had a full initial clinical assessment, tests were only performed when further information was required to assist in diagnosis, prognosis or treatment. It was fundamental to good medical practice to avoid subjecting the patient to the inconvenience and risks of unnecessary interventions, and adding unnecessary costs. 'Routine' investigations lead to a hit-and-miss approach. They can provide equivocal results which add further to diagnostic problems, to confusion, poor clinical practice to the patient's time on the medical treadmill. Tests can also be ably abetted by the influence of the medical industry and in some cases can be related to the vested interest of doctors and hospitals.

The access to modern methods of investigation has added substantially to our ability to diagnose and to treat patients with heart disease. These tests include imaging techniques such as echocardiography, MRI and angiography. In many patients these investigations are appropriate and essential in practice but it is inevitable that the increasing reliance on tests could lead to a decline in clinical practice and even in the vital contact between doctor and patient, as it can be damaging to the counselling role of the doctor. Clinical evaluation through the seeking-out of symptoms and examination of the patient should remain the bedrock of good medical practice. In most cases simply listening to your patient will tell you what is wrong

Some doctors will argue that they must do tests to avoid medical litigation. However, litigation is highly unlikely to succeed if it is shown that a proper clinical evaluation was carried out, nor are patients who have close contact with their doctor so likely to proceed to court. The current exponential increase in the cost of our health service and in those in other western countries will continue as the march of high-tech medicine continues, particularly among colleagues who fail to establish a satisfactory professional relationship with their patients. It needs to be said that most doctors today retain their clinical skills and are selective in their choice of investigations, but for others the routine performance of tests is leading to a culture of practice which is undesirable.

6

THE RISE AND FALL OF THE CORONARY EPIDEMIC

Coronary heart disease is a general term to include disturbances of heart function and structure caused by interference with the blood supply to the heart muscle. The heart muscle is highly specialised, designed to remain active during a person's whole lifetime, and the heart rate responds to exercise and other physiological activities, such as stress and digestion, by increasing in rate to increase the blood supply to the body, including its own muscle, and to provide more oxygen for active muscles and other active processes. The heart is fist-sized and its muscle is unlike the muscles we use for our normal daily activities. It is in a constant state of activity, contracting and relaxing about every second of one's life. This regular cyclical activity is maintained by a small area of specialised muscle cells in the right upper chamber of the heart (the right atrium), which sparks off an impulse every second or so and sends an electro-chemical message along special pathways that initiates contraction of the muscle cells in all parts of the organ.

Heart muscle function is dependent on the supply of blood that reaches it through the coronary arteries. The supply of oxygen and the removal of the products of metabolism, such as carbon dioxide, are dependent on this active blood supply, which can vary in volume in response to the needs of the living tissues. If the heart muscle is suddenly deprived of its blood supply, its regular contraction and relaxation may break down and stop functioning within a matter of seconds. Even if part of the muscle is affected, it may cause the entire muscle to malfunction, leading to the same result.

Coronary heart disease is a major cause of ill health and premature death in Ireland and other western countries. It is a manmade disease in the sense that it is provoked by factors in our environment and because of our western lifestyles. The causes are now well known, but until they were identified by epidemiological research into populations during the last fifty years and the appropriate lifestyle changes were encouraged, we were helpless in dealing with the gathering epidemic in the mid-twentieth century.

Reviewing the exciting period of clinical practice and research I enjoyed during my active career, I would say that the greatest contribution we made in my hospital was the emphasis we placed on the causes of disease: identifying the risk factor and, encouraging smokers to quit and promoting high blood pressure control, healthy nutrition and encouraging aerobic physical activity. This lifestyle approach was both logical and rational in preventing and treating the disease although the medical profession as a whole and at an international level was slow to introduce this preventive approach. It is only in the recent past that prevention became part of medical and hospital practice and that the importance of rehabilitation of patients who suffer from coronary disease became widely appreciated. There had been a poor commitment to prevention and health promotion and a lack of attention to causes within the profession, both in training and in practice. Indeed, much still has to be done in this area. Neglect by the profession has been shared by our politicians, who could do much more to encourage a healthier society.

My interest in epidemiology, the study of disease in populations, stems from the late 1950s when I first began to see increasing numbers of patients with coronary heart disease as the epidemic was gathering. It came upon on us like a thief in the night. I became curious about the cause of the sudden epidemic. Indeed, my interest started earlier, when I adopted a programme of smoking cessation and graduated walking exercise for patients with the related arterial disease of the legs. I was committed as a student to cardiology when I read the third edition of Paul White's 1944 textbook, *Heart Disease*, and later in London with my interest in disease of the leg vessels. White had done much clinical research into coronary disease and he was the first to publish a full and rational review of the pathological link between atherosclerosis, the disease in the coronary arteries, and angina and heart attacks. He underlined the frequency of disease in the coronary vessels in patients with these conditions. It was to take many more years before this link and the basis of the coronary epidemic was to be accepted by the general medical profession, and even longer to identify the causes of atherosclerosis and coronary disease. During my student and resident years at St Vincent's from 1942–1946, there was little conception among my physician teachers about the pathology, natural history and clinical features of coronary heart disease, nor was there any knowledge of its epidemiology and causation. Indeed it was to take many more years after the Second World War for many practitioners to understand the nature and full significance of coronary disease and the coronary epidemic.

White was later to become an advocate of heart disease prevention and was critical of the many forms of treatment advocated by doctors without proper evidence of efficacy. He was one of a few physicians who established the American Heart Association and encouraged the heart association movement in other countries. He encouraged epidemiological research into heart disease in the United States after the Second World War. Famous as Eisenhower's doctor after the President's heart attack, he was an advocate of health promotion, including healthy eating, weight control and exercise. He was a step ahead of his colleagues with his initiatives and insights and often brought the fight for prevention into the realm of politics. White attended the launch of the Irish Heart Foundation in 1966 and later I was sent by him to organise a heart foundation in Greece, but this proved to be a difficult task; it is almost beyond the ability of a simple Irishman to unravel the politics of some of our continental colleagues. Eventually, Greece did acquire its own foundation but only after a number of years and much infighting. I visited White on a few occasions, including an address I gave to the Boston Medical Society recalling Corrigan, Stokes, Graves and other famous Irish physicians of the nineteenth century. It was his custom to insist that his visitors should mow his lawn during visits to his house and I was one of his willing victims!

My interest in epidemiology has given me insights into clinical medicine of which I would otherwise have been unaware. In particular, it has stimulated my interest in causation and in the understanding of the natural history of disease. The coronary epidemic peaked in Ireland in the 1960s and early 1970s. By then a persistent decline began with a fall of coronary deaths of up to 70 percent by 2008, particularly among the middle aged. Cigarette smoking had also changed during this time: more than 60 percent of adult males were smokers in the 1960s but this fell to 24 percent by 2005 and by this date the greatest decline in smoking was among the older age groups, who were at the highest risk. Important changes in eating habits and better blood pressure control have also benefited public health over the past forty years; heart-related deaths in all western countries are falling and converging. All-cause mortality has declined to the lowest level in the history of the State, thanks largely to the fall in coronary and stroke mortality.

The dramatic decline of coronary disease has been studied by groups of cardiologists, economists, statisticians and epidemiologists in Ireland and several other countries. All of these studies agree that the decline in coronary disease can be attributed mostly to lifestyle changes. They are consistent in finding that reduction in cigarette smoking alone accounts on average for 45 percent of the lower mortality, while coronary surgery accounts for less than 3 percent of the decline. These findings have been reported by me in detail in the *Irish Medical Journal* in February 2006.

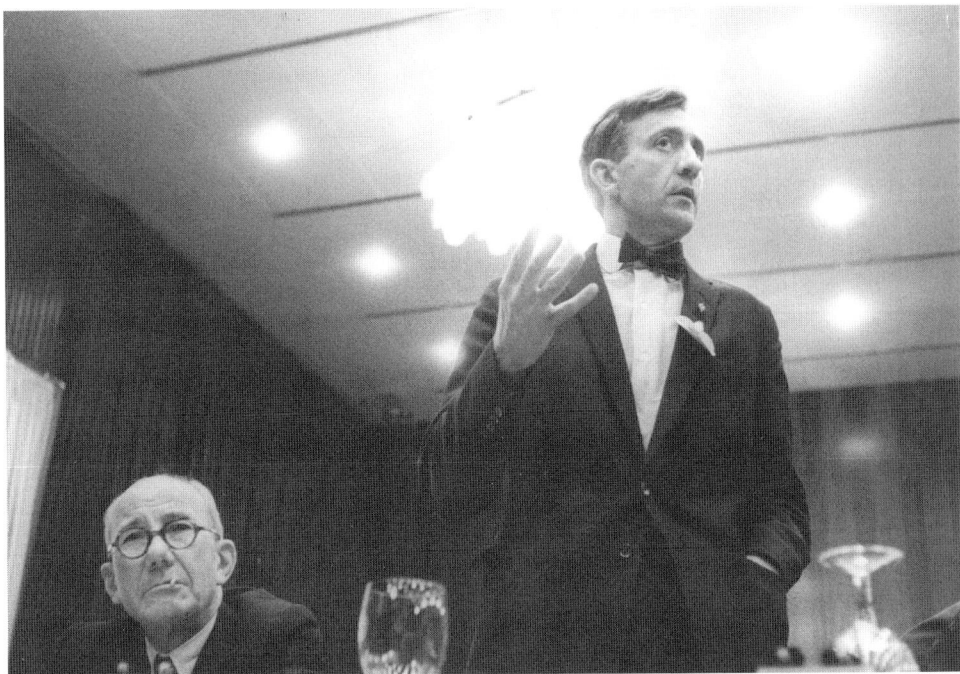

Addressing the conference of the European Society of Cardiology

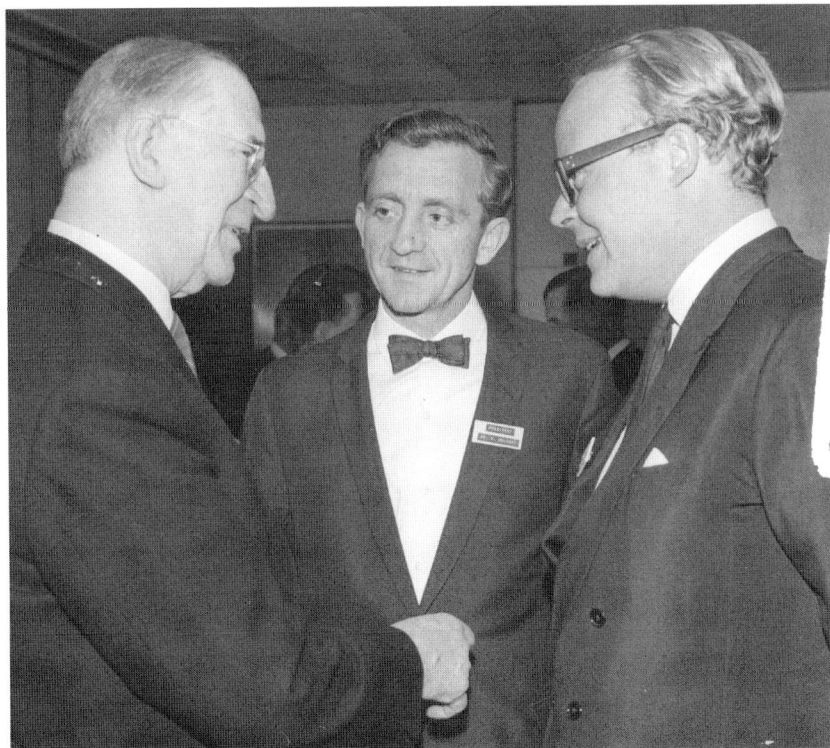

At the launch of the Irish Heart Foundation in 1966 with Eamon de Valera and Benjamin Guinness, Lord Iveagh, the honorary treasurer of the IHF

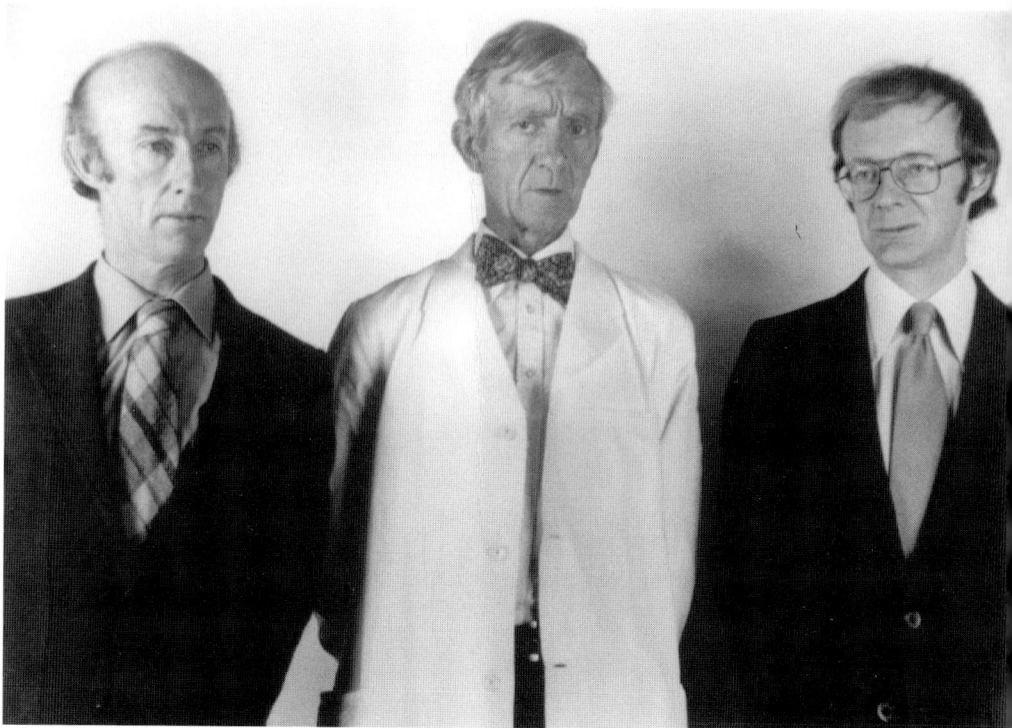

The St Vincent's Hospital research team, 1981: Noel Hickey, author and Ian Graha

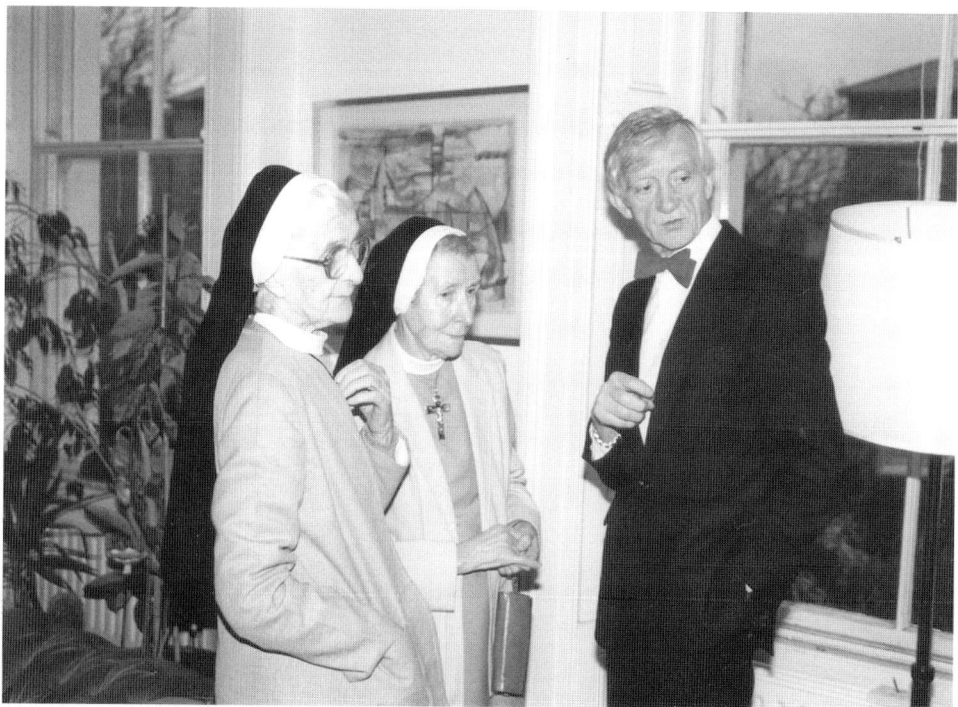

Author with Sisters Padua and Paul at St Vincent's Hospital

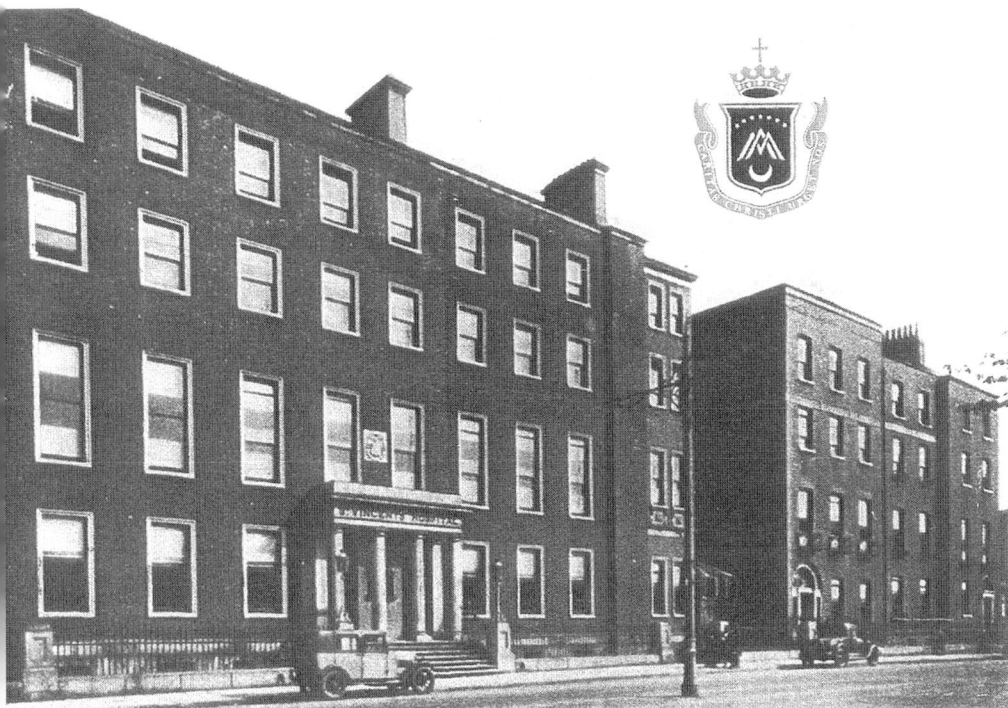

St Vincent's Hospital at St Stephen's Green in the 1920s. The crest *caritas Christi urget nos* ('The charity of Christ inspires us') is the precept of the Sisters of Charity, who established the Order and the hospital in 1834

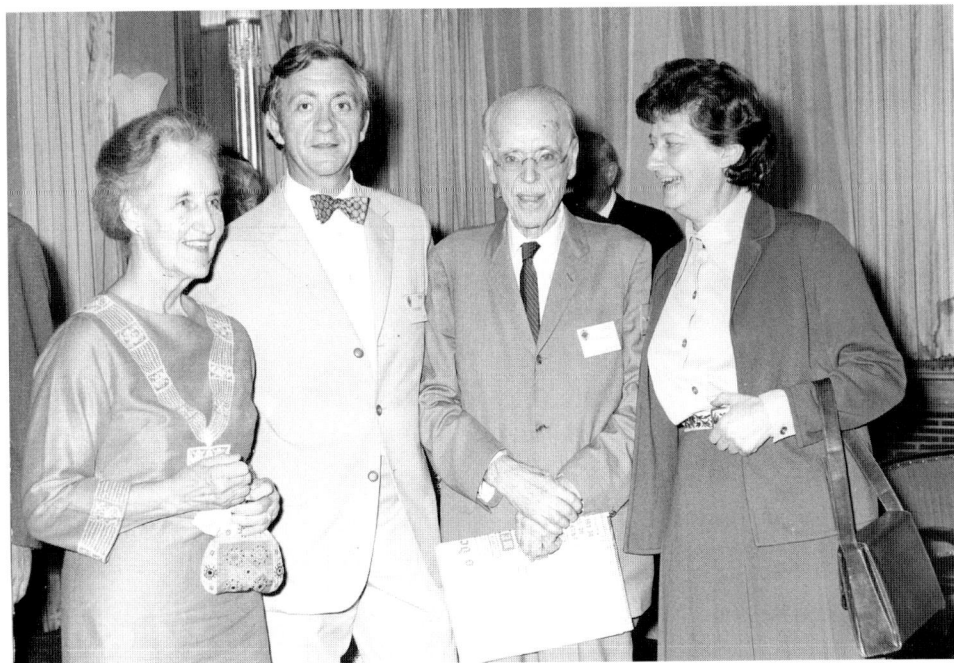

At the 1970 World Congress of Cardiology, in London. From left: Helen White, author, Paul White and Rose Stamler

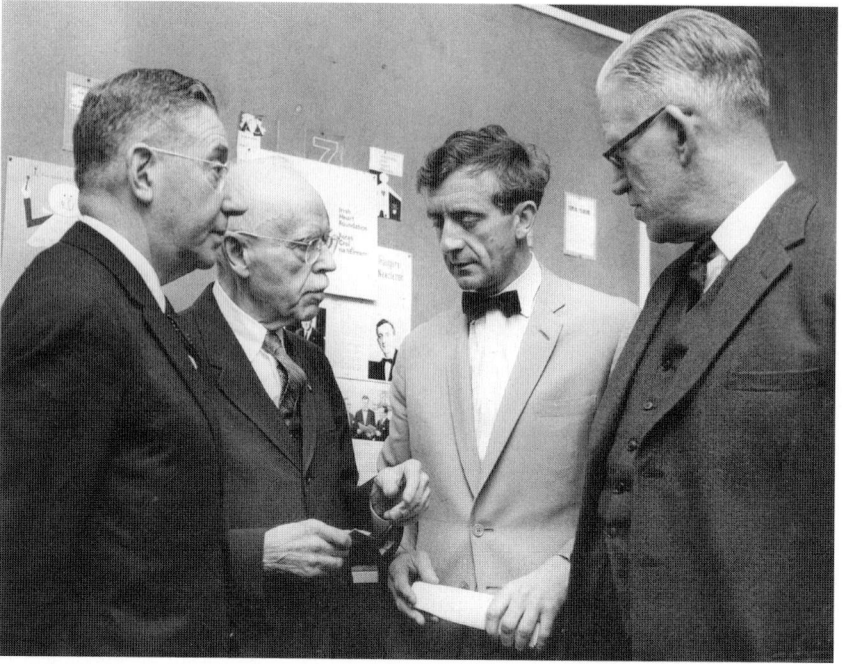

At the launch of the Irish Heart Foundation. From left: Albert Baer of New York, Paul White, author and Graham Hayward, president of the British Heart Foundation

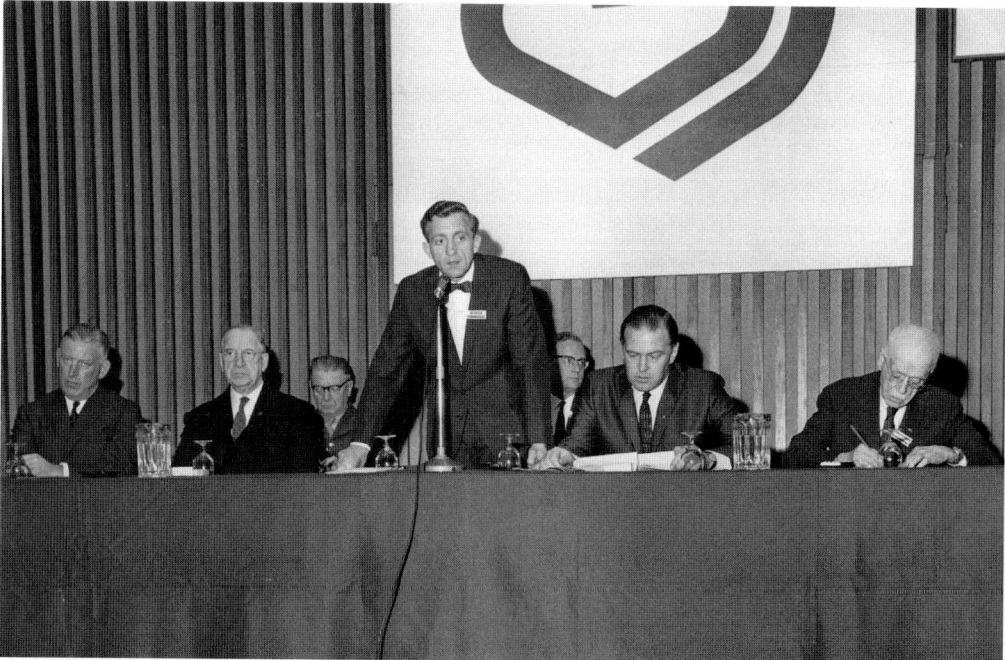

At the same event. From left: Graham Hayward, Eamon de Valera, author, Donnacha O'Malley and Paul White

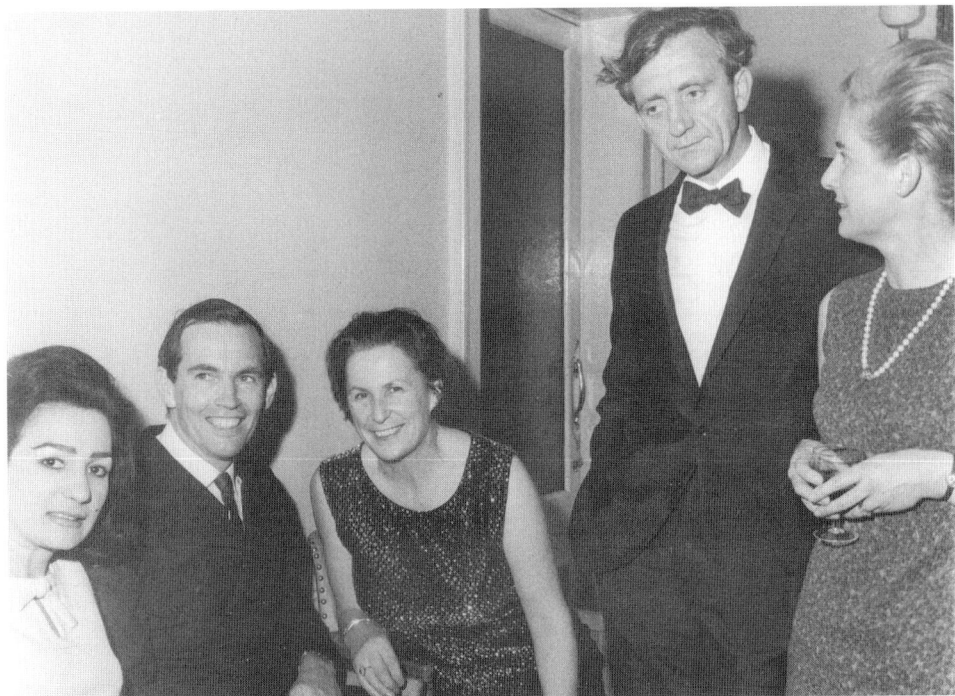

Maria Dean, Christiaan Barnard (who performed the world's first successful heart transplant), Fanty O'Dwyer, author and Peg Towers, *c.* 1971

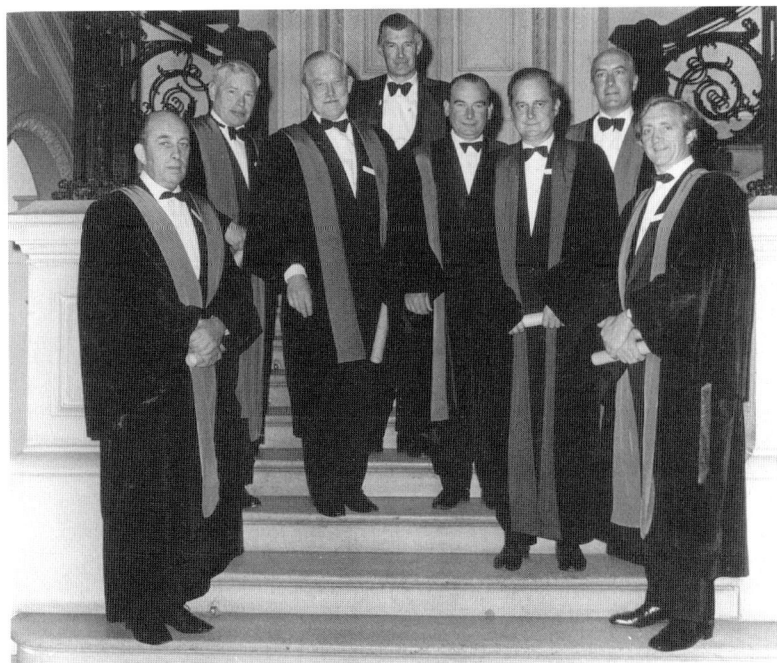

With colleagues, being admitted as fellows of the Royal College of Physicians in Ireland, 1973

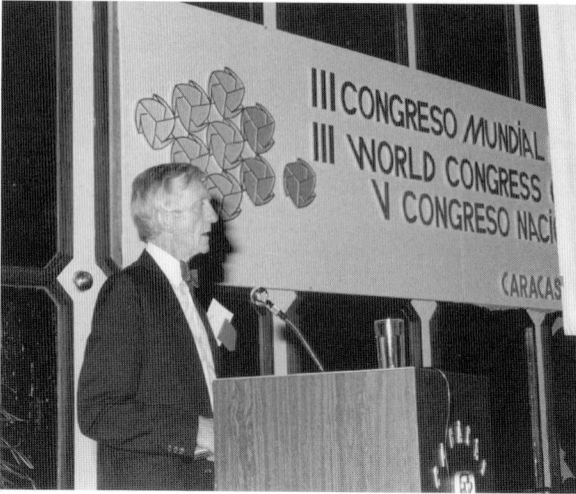

Addressing the World
Congress of Cardiology
in Venezuela, 1990

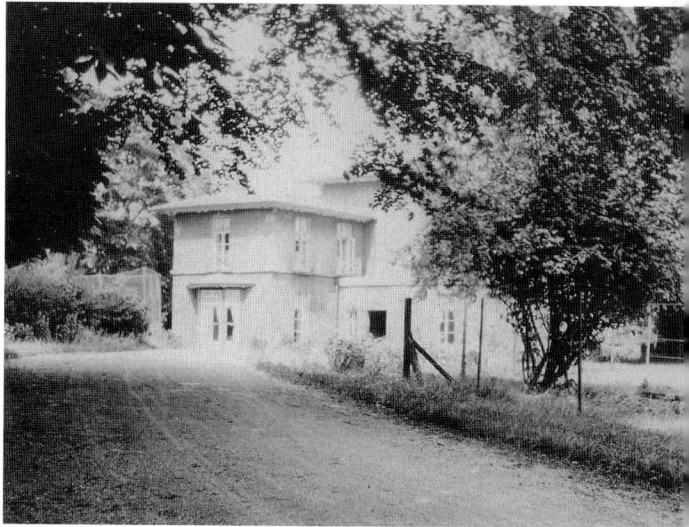

Lissenfield House, 1923

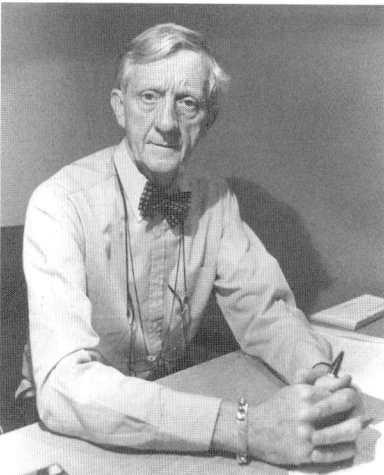

Portrait, 1990

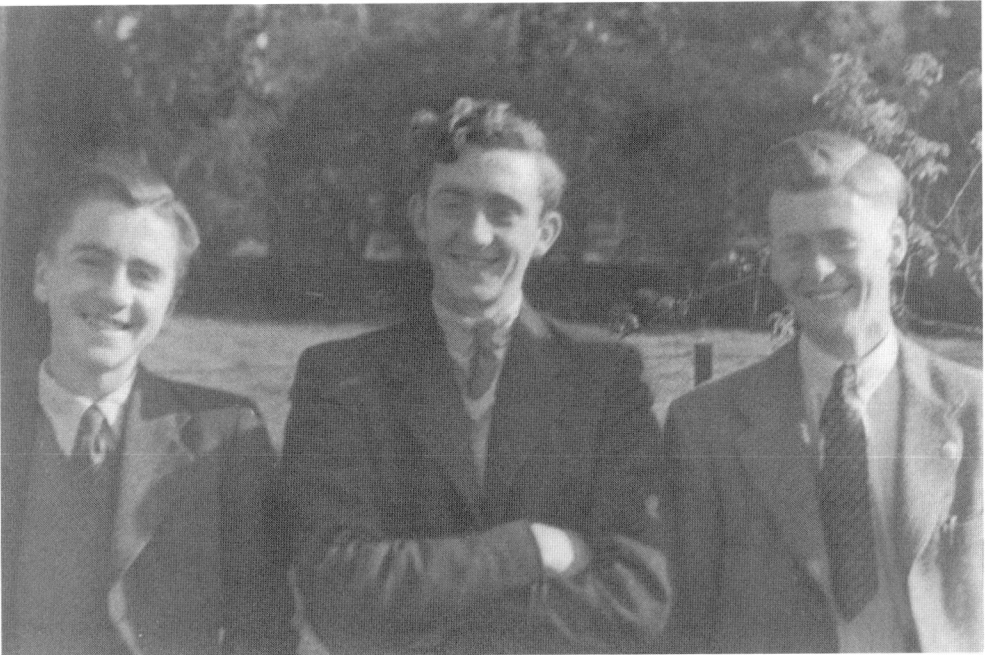

With my brothers, Seán (left) and Pádraig (right)

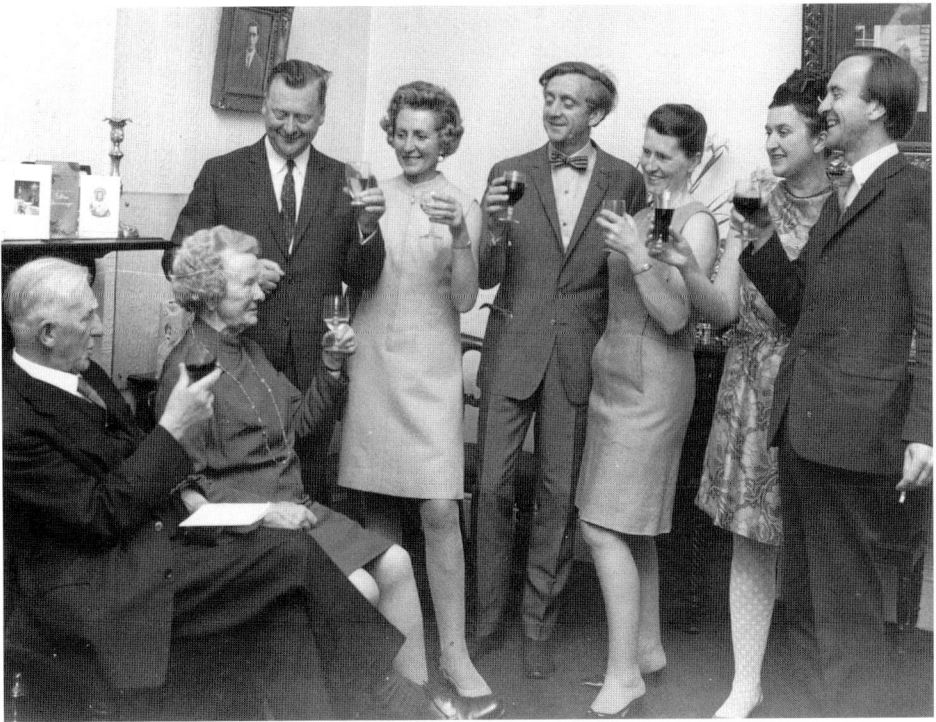

At my parents' fiftieth anniversary, 1969. From left: Pádraig, Elisabet, author, Máire, Neillí and Seán

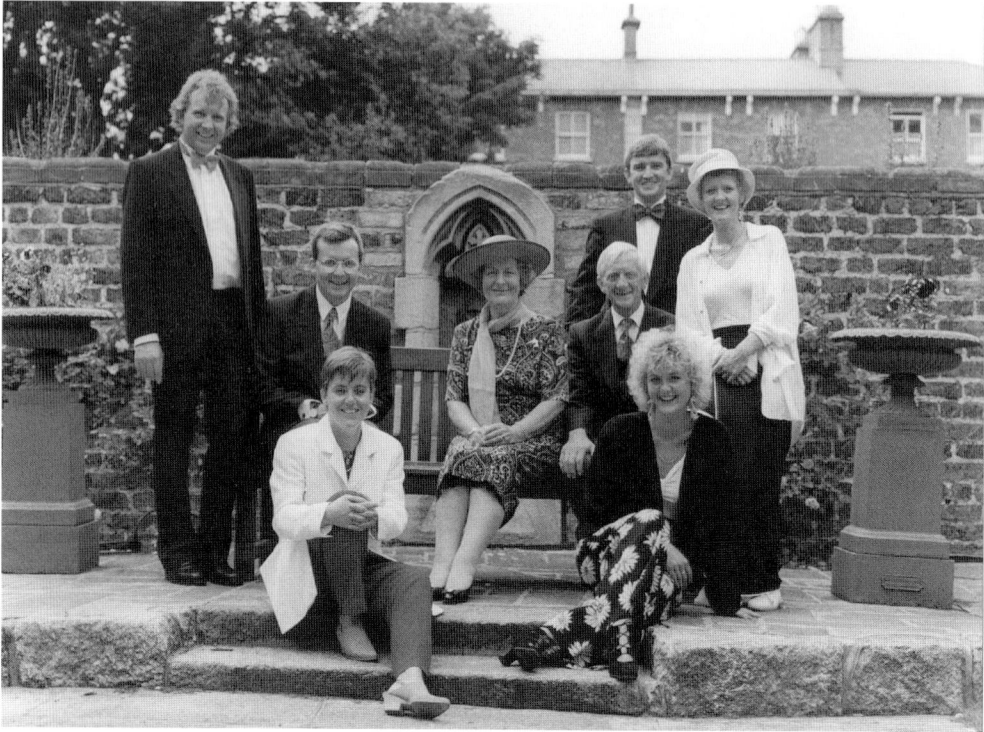

With my first wife, Aileen (centre), and children at the Berkeley Court Hotel, Dublin, on the occasion of my son Hugh's wedding to Martha Ellison in 1994. Left: Richard, Hugh and Lisa (seated). Right: David, Tina and Barbara (seated)

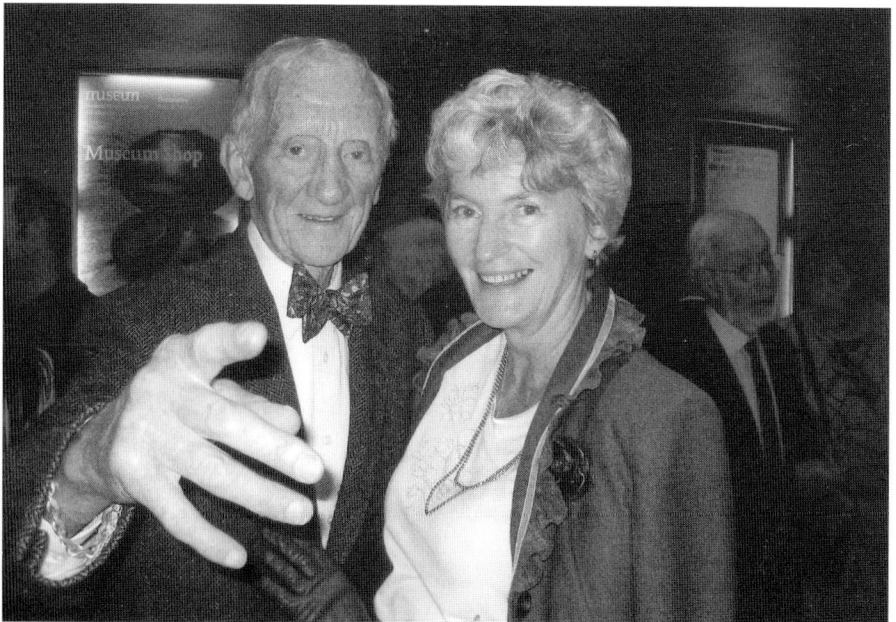

With my wife, Louise Hederman

7

ATHEROSCLEROSIS AND CORONARY HEART DISEASE

Disease of the coronary arteries, called atherosclerosis (from the Greek *athero* = chaff or porridge; *sklerosis* = hardening) is the basis of coronary heart disease and its various manifestations, and may be present without causing symptoms. Here I use the term 'coronary artery disease'; the term 'coronary heart disease' indicates that the disease presents itself in clinical form because it has reached the stage of causing a temporary or permanent interference with the blood supply to part of the heart muscle.

Many adults in modern western society have some disease in one or more coronary arteries without being aware of it. They complain of no subjective symptoms and no objective clinical signs will be evident to the examining doctor. It is generally only when the disease is more advanced or it becomes more unstable that it leads to interference with blood flow, and to an appreciable reduction in the blood supply to the affected part of the muscle. Atherosclerosis presents as an irregular thickening of the inner lining of the artery, which may lead to significant partial or complete blockages and which, when advanced, may lead to significant reduction in or to a total obstruction of blood supply to the heart. The three coronary arteries are fairly constant in their distribution around the human heart.

The diseased tissue in the arteries is made up of various constituents, including cholesterol, and it is the location, the rate of onset and the severity of the atherosclerotic process that determine the onset of coronary heart disease. Cholesterol is one of a number of fats which are normally present in the human body. It is formed in the liver from fats absorbed from food and is an essential part of the human cell which serves a number of other functions which are fundamental to life, reproduction and human health. Disturbances of cholesterol metabolism are the basis of disease of the arteries.

The presence of atherosclerosis in the arteries has been noted since the beginning of modern history. It has been found in Egyptian mummies and was noted by medieval physicians when post-mortem examinations were first carried out. However, its nature has only been recognised since the nineteenth century, when its rich content of cholesterol and other signs of degeneration and healing were described by some of the great pathologists of that time. There is little doubt that the different clinical manifestations of coronary heart disease occurred in the distant past, if one is to judge by the frequent references to sudden death (often attributed to stroke or poisoning); and deaths associated with chest pain, although their causes were not understood.

Of course, effective treatment of any condition must depend on knowledge of causation; and every disease has a physical cause. If we know the cause, we can generally prevent the disease. The elimination of causes in healthy patients is called 'primary prevention'. Elimination of complications and further attacks in a patient already afflicted by disease is called 'secondary prevention', and is again dependent on understanding causes.

The progress of atherosclerosis and its complications can be retarded or reversed, but only if it is treated as a chronic condition and over the long term. This does not necessarily require long-term dependence on doctors but it needs more than simply dealing with the acute event alone. The affected patient must adopt lifestyle changes which are known to improve the long-term prognosis by preventing the accumulation of atherosclerosis, by stabilising the artery lining, and by reducing further acute events. It is treatment aimed at prevention through risk factor intervention, an approach which has been neglected by the profession while there has been an excessive over reliance on drugs, coronary surgery and angioplasty.

Doctors should therefore be concerned about the causes of atherosclerosis as well as the precipitating factors that can lead to the initial symptoms or sudden heart attack. The fundamental approach should aim to prevent atherosclerosis at a primary level, which has been the objective of many organisations, including our own research and the Irish Heart Foundation, during the last forty years.

Atherosclerosis affects many of the arteries of the body. The main arteries to the brain, the carotid vessels, and their branches are also prone to atherosclerosis, where blockages may lead to temporary neurological symptoms called transient ischaemic attacks. These blockages are also a major cause of stroke with the cutting off of the blood supply to important parts of the brain. Like a patient admitted with a heart attack, if a stroke victim is seen quickly after the onset of the attack, the blockage in the artery can be dissolved or bypassed.

Atherosclerosis is common in the leg vessels, leading to a symptom called intermittent claudication, a syndrome simulating angina of effort where the patient may develop severe muscle pain due to insufficient oxygen supply while walking or otherwise exerting the legs. If the disease process in the leg vessels is severe it may lead to a critically reduced circulation to the legs and prolonged pain while at rest or the permanent cutting-off of blood supply, causing gangrene and requiring amputation. Atherosclerosis is not uncommon in the main blood vessel of the body, the aorta, which extends from the heart and through its main branches supplies the head, neck, body, arms and lower limbs. The atherosclerotic process in the aorta may lead to serious obstruction at the exit of some of its main branches. It may also lead to such damage to the wall of the artery that it may distend like a balloon and eventually rupture. This we describe as an aneurysm, not an uncommon finding in older people prone to atherosclerotic disease.

Angina of effort is one of the most frequent clinical symptoms of coronary heart disease and has been recognised for many years. The most celebrated case was that of the famous British surgeon John Hunter who lived in London in the late eighteenth century and who described the symptom in his famous book *A treatise on the blood, inflammation and gun-shot wounds* (1794). He described how his own chest pain was caused by emotional upset induced by conflict with his colleagues. His description was very clear-cut but the true nature of his problem was not known at that time. Not unexpectedly, he died suddenly during an altercation.

When the blockage is more significant, the angina may become more severe or the patient may have a heart attack, leading to heart muscle damage called myocardial infarction (Greek: *myo* = muscle, *cardiac* = heart; Latin: *infarc* = stuffed), previously called coronary thrombosis. The extent of heart muscle damage depends on the size and location of the blocked vessel and to a lesser extent on the presence of a collateral circulation.

The diagnosis of myocardial infarction and its relation with coronary artery disease was first precisely described in 1912 by an American physician but the link was not understood by the profession until after the Second World when it was finally accepted by cardiologists in Britain, Ireland and the United States. However, the widespread acceptance of myocardial infarction and its underlying pathology took at least another twenty or thirty years to be widely accepted and not confused with other clinical conditions. As late as the 1960s, the newspapers in Ireland were reporting that patients who had died suddenly of a myocardial infarction had died from acute indigestion, and even doctors often misclassified them as having died from strokes or other causes, including such fanciful condition as *status lymphaticus* (a meaningless Latin term to conceal our ignorance) and divine intervention!

The treatment of myocardial infarction has greatly improved in recent years, but to be effective in patients at the acute stage they need to be seen and admitted immediately after onset of symptoms to an appropriate facility in hospital. Going back twenty-five years or more, our hospital coronary register confirmed a mortality rate in patients admitted with a myocardial infarction of about 12 percent. Today in the coronary units the mortality has been more than halved thanks to new treatment methods which are designed to dissolve the underlying clotting in the artery. Even without treatment, many patients will still survive unless the heart damage is extensive or unless the attack leads to ventricular fibrillation and sudden death. Most of the sudden, unexpected deaths in the Western World are the result of sudden clotting and myocardial infarction.

In those who survive the attack, their future progress is largely determined by the extent of residual heart muscle damage. Many patients do survive and return to normal living after the heart muscle has healed, which happens within a few weeks. They may experience no further trouble, particularly if they follow appropriate lifestyle and medical advice. Those who survive with extensive damage may take longer to recover and tend to have less favourable early prognoses than those with less damage. However, in my clinical and research experience, if they survive the first year or two, with proper rehabilitation and management they can do equally as well in the long run as those with less damage.

During a coronary attack sudden death is not uncommon. The cause is a breakdown in the electro-chemical conduction system of the heart called ventricular fibrillation. The heart can no longer function and the human brain can only endure survival for about three minutes if it is deprived of its blood supply at normal body temperature. Almost invariably the patient will be brain dead within that short time, unless cardio-respiratory resuscitation and defibrillation are performed immediately. Sudden death, often accompanied by chest and arm pain, was a common feature of life in the 1950s and 1960s and was a frequent event in the home, in the community, on golf courses and at football matches. The mechanism of such sudden death was not fully understood even by trained cardiologists until the early 1960s, although we were perfectly aware that it was related to disease of the coronary arteries. It was not until the development of the visual display unit and the visual demonstration of heart rhythms which it provided that the concept of ventricular fibrillation was established as by far the most common cause of sudden death. This discovery, combined with electric defibrillation of the heart and the contemporary development of a practical form of cardio-respiratory resuscitation (CPR) introduced the concept of coronary care.

A Dr Wiggers in the United States in 1915 was the first to describe ventricular fibrillation on a dog, whose heartbeat he returned to normal by administering an electric shock. He confirmed the diagnosis by the fine movements of fibrillation and the inert heart in the dog's open chest. This concept was first put into practice in the 1960s and became a widespread facility relatively quickly in all of our general hospitals.

8

HEART RESEARCH AT ST VINCENT'S HOSPITAL

By the late 1950s, Dr Ancel Keyes of Minneapolis, Minnesota in the United States, in the ambitious and inspired 'Seven Countries' study, had identified a high incidence of coronary disease in those countries where the population had high blood cholesterol levels. The rationale of his research was based on the well-known presence of cholesterol in the atherosclerotic plaque. He also confirmed that populations with high levels of cholesterol in their diet had a higher saturated fat intake. This is the fat found in meat of domestic animals, in dairy foods and certain other sources. Other studies in the United States at that time were also including cholesterol as part of their research work into coronary disease. However, it was to take many more years, and the opposition of a conservative profession and of the food and dairy industries, before the importance of cholesterol and saturated fat were to be accepted as major factors in the genesis of coronary disease.

The identification of the causes of coronary heart disease was achieved in a relatively short period, starting in about the mid-1950s when Ancel Keys set up the Seven Countries study. About the same time a few major epidemiological studies were established in the United States, which carried out research at two levels: the prospective population studies on the one hand and clinical case history, or 'cohort studies', on the other.

Prospective studies were considered the more reliable means of identifying causes (soon to be called 'risk factors'), but they had the disadvantage of being very expensive, in most cases costing several million dollars during their lifetime. It is obvious therefore why these studies were first organised in a wealthy country such as the United States, where the coronary epidemic presented earliest and in its most virulent form. Prospective studies required a relatively large permanent staff trained in epidemiological methods of recording, evaluation and interpretation; and needed some years to arrive at reliable and incontrovertible results. The Seven Countries study, the Framingham study in Boston, the Tecumseh study in Cleveland, and the Hammond and Horn group in California were some of these. They eventually showed considerable agreement in confirming the causes of cardiac disease.

In these studies large numbers of apparently healthy people were included initially to determine their various baseline physical, social and psychological characteristics. They were followed up for ten years or more to determine the association of such characteristics with the subsequent development of disease. The prospective studies produced a huge amount of information, not only about the causes of coronary artery disease, stroke and related conditions, but also about cancer and other chronic conditions. By the late 1960s, it was becoming more apparent that abnormal cholesterol metabolism was a basic contributing factor and that coronary disease was commonest in those who smoked cigarettes, who had higher blood pressure and who performed less aerobic exercise.

The other method of research was the case history approach. Here, the subjects were patients already suffering from the disease. This method of enquiry had the great advantage of requiring a much smaller number of subjects, of being much less expensive than the prospective studies and of being carried out during the patient's treatment in hospital. The cohort study was considered less satisfactory by the international cardiovascular epidemiologists with whom I worked, but few of them were practising clinicians and I did not agree with most of their reservations. Later, I published a paper in the *Irish Journal of Medical Science* on the advantages and merits of the case history approach.

It was the case history method of research which I adopted, because it could be done as part of my ordinary day-to-day practice in my newly acquired department of sixteen beds. Initially, it required no special staff and only the expenses were associated with recording and retrieving information. Research was ongoing during my time at St Vincent's but did not require massive additional funding for a great increase in staff. In later years when our research work was in full flight we managed with four full-time research workers, as well as my colleague Noel Hickey, who was also attached to the University's department of preventive medicine, and Ian Graham as a senior research fellow for five years. There were other part-time contributors including a statistician and a psychologist.

By adopting the strictest principles of evidence, the epidemiologist laid the groundwork for effective research into the ills of western society. We were heavily dependent of the services of the statistician. The medical statistician was an essential member of the research and training group to ensure that conclusions about cause and effect were justified and that all confounding influences were recognised. The epidemiologists were remarkable for their strict adherence to principles which demanded that evidence be based on concrete grounds.

Within a much shorter timeframe and for a fraction of the expense of a prospective study, a properly designed case history study could provide sufficient information about causation to influence patient management and to give guidelines about primary and secondary prevention. When the patients are followed up afterwards, as in the St Vincent's study where follow-up was extended for forty-one years (along the lines of the prospective studies), an immense amount of new knowledge can – and did – accrue. That is not to say that the prospective studies could be dispensed with. They were essential in confirming other approaches to research, and their results were necessary to convince a conservative profession and influence a public largely ignorant in matters of health. It was the prospective studies which, because of their wide publicity and reflection of the results of clinical studies such as ours, which were to have the greatest influence on the profession and the public.

There had been a few case history studies in the United States after 1940 about the high prevalence of smoking among coronary patients, but little notice was taken of these. Little credence was given to the relationship between smoking and coronary disease, even by the Royal College of Physicians report on smoking and health in 1963 and the Surgeon General of the United States in his seminal first report in 1964. The main emphasis in these two reports was on cigarette smoking, lung cancer and respiratory disease. There were also occasional murmurings that patients with high blood pressure might be more prone to heart attack, but little attention was paid to this factor in these early years.

I first added research into the rehabilitation of coronary patients and epidemiology to my role as a clinical doctor in the early 1960s. Medical epidemiology is the study of disease in populations and is aimed at studying social and cultural factors which provide information on causes. In the realm of the chronic diseases, it is not possible to identify causes at the bedside or during surgery because causes cannot be separated easily from confounding factors and individual patients differ widely in characteristics and social backgrounds. Without the benefits of population studies or the careful collection of adequate data during a case history study, it would have been difficult to acquire the knowledge we have about the lifestyle changes which have led to the dramatic decline in mortality from heart disease. Epidemiological studies are the lifeblood of prevention. The most vocal critics of our advocacy of lifestyle changes based on epidemiological studies were those doctors who had little knowledge of the potential of epidemiological research in exploring and understanding the nature of the chronic diseases

Rehabilitation is aimed at returning a patient to a normal life after recovery from an illness and preventing further complications or recurrences of the disease. We have learned from epidemiological studies that the same lifestyle changes which prevent disease in the healthy population are also effective in reducing recurrence in patients already afflicted by disease. Such secondary prevention is a crucial part of management of coronary patients.

The five years from 1961–1966 were probably the most difficult and traumatic of my career. Coronary heart disease had reached epidemic proportions, with some patients as young as thirty or forty years of age suffering and dying from the disease. Most were men, but there were some women, and virtually all the younger victims were smokers. Until 1966 and the setting up of our coronary care unit in June of that year, there was little we could do to deal with the complications which were all too common among coronary patients.

It was the immediate problems arising during the acute stage which were the greatest source of difficulty. Sudden death amongst the acute cases was common. We did not understand why the heart stopped in some patients and not in others. All too often, before establishing the coronary care unit, I would get urgent calls, day or night, weekday or weekend, if a patient developed symptoms of acute heart failure, recurring heart pain and particularly if the patient died suddenly. My constant attendances on such patients were not only disruptive in terms of my daily life, but my inability to deal with many of the complications was both frustrating and traumatic. I remember a few instances particularly.

A thirty-eight-year-old son of a close friend of the family was admitted to our private nursing home and appeared to make a good recovery after an acute heart attack. On the fourth or fifth day, I received an urgent call and on arriving found he was dead. Another time, I was called to a forty-year-old foreign doctor who appeared to be having a heart attack. I arrived quickly at his small flat and found him lying on a stretcher bed. He was warm, but dead. His wife and three young children were there. I went through the then-newly described procedure of cardio-respiratory resuscitation, but every time I pressed his chest to maintain heart function, his heavy frame just sank deeper into the stretcher bed. I knew perfectly well that he was beyond resuscitation but I went through the procedure with the wife leaning over my shoulder saying to me again and again, 'Will he be alright doctor? Will he be alright?' Eventually I stopped my futile efforts at resuscitation and told her quite clearly that he was dead and that there was nothing I could do except send for an ambulance. She found it impossible to comprehend the tragedy and held on tightly to me repeating, 'Well, will he be all right?' I think that it was one of the most desperate and lonely situations I ever remember.

I was called urgently one evening to see a middle-aged patient in Mullingar; I attended him with his local practitioner. He had a severe pain in his chest and had clearly developed a myocardial infarction but his chest pain subsided before I arrived and he appeared to be reasonably comfortable. After I took his history and examined him, I did what was customary; I retired to another room with his doctor to discuss his case.

Having discussed his case we then had the relatives join us and I explained to them that he appeared to have had a full heart attack but that he had settled down, was now more comfortable and that he should remain there until the following day when an ambulance would take him up to my hospital. As was also customary, we returned to the patient's room to explain the situation to him. He was dead. I went through the process of pummelling his chest, but this was before we had learnt the technique of cardio-respiratory resuscitation. Anyhow, there was little I could have done and I hardly need say how traumatised I felt on the occasion. I stayed on for some considerable length of time with the family and eventually retired to the doctor's house where a glass or two of whisky and some coffee were sufficient to restore my morale and to keep me awake on my way home.

In the early years of practice, before the availability of specialists in provincial hospitals, I was frequently called to see country patients who were acutely ill. Not all calls were as traumatic as those I've just described. I was called to see a seventy-five-year-old man on one occasion by a practitioner friend of mine about seventy miles from Dublin. The patient was semi-conscious having suffered a severe stroke. I pronounced him to be dying and beyond treatment. In discussing the case with his doctor afterwards, I said, 'What in the name of God did you expect me to do when the patient was obviously moribund?' He replied that it was important that the relatives should be satisfied that all was being done for their loved one. A few months later we met at a meeting of the Irish Medical Association in Killarney. He was a larger than life character and a long-standing friend. As I walked into the crowded bar of the Europa Hotel, he was there and on seeing me shouted in the presence of all our colleagues, 'Risteárd, you remember the man you saw last November in Thurles who you said was dying and beyond help? Well I played nine holes with him at the weekend!'

Because of our relative helplessness in those early days, and the frequency of heart attacks and sudden death, even among those in early middle age, it is understandable that my physician colleagues at St Vincent's Hospital were reluctant to look after such patients and that I was encouraged by them to take sole charge of all coronary admissions. This may appear to have been a poisoned chalice or at least a mixed blessing, but it proved to be providential. Until 1960 I was nominally a junior physician with an official complement of two beds and with busy out-patient duties, although I had been appointed nine years before as a cardiologist. I soon found my position in the hospital more appropriate when I was provided with a custom-built sixteen-bed unit which afterwards was to prove ideal for a coronary care facility.

During a two-month fellowship which brought me to the United States in early 1962, I was fortunate to meet most of the leading American cardiovascular epidemiologists and I travelled to the major research centres which were in the early stages of their population research. Ancel Keys and Henry Blackburn of Minneapolis, Jeremiah Stamler and his wife, Rose, of Chicago, Fred Epstein of Cleveland, and William Kannell of Framingham and others. These four groups had already set up major prospective population studies in response to the mounting coronary epidemic in the US. Prospective studies were based on studying large numbers of healthy people to identify many physical, social, occupational and psychological factors which might provide clues to the causes of common diseases like coronary disease.

We at St Vincent's had commenced our own study of patients admitted with heart attacks in 1961 and the American visit was hugely encouraging in our research into the characteristics of our coronary patients. In our case history study, we used the 'Cope Chat' system of data collection and information retrieval. Before the arrival of computers, with this simple but effective method we were able to record and retrieve eighty clinical, social, behavioural, and psychological characteristics and attributes of all our patients admitted with confirmed heart attacks.

Within two years we identified the high prevalence of cigarette smoking, high blood pressure and abnormal blood cholesterol patterns among our patients compared with healthy controls in the normal population. We published papers in the national and international medical journals about the risk profiles of both women and men. Apart from the numerous male patients, we recorded detailed information on about a hundred women younger than sixty who had had heart attacks and found that their risk factors were the same as men's. This paper was published in the American heart journal *Circulation* in 1967 and was, as far as I could ascertain, the first paper to be published on risk factors in women with coronary disease. Women were just as prone to coronary disease as men, but smoked little at the time in Ireland and other western counties, and had more normal cholesterol profiles. Hence they had a lower prevalence of the disease.

In early 1965 we commenced a long-term follow-up study of carefully selected male patients less than sixty years who had survived a first heart attack by one month. Eleven years later, by December 1975, we had included 555 successive subjects who satisfied the strict criteria of the study. They were the group which provided the material for our future studies into heart disease. All patients were seen three times during the first year after discharge and then once every subsequent year. The last follow up was completed in the autumn of 2006, forty-one years later. Thus, we combined a follow-up study with our case-history material. Thirty of these subjects were still alive at the end of 2006 and only ten were unavailable for follow-up, some because of residence abroad.

Our follow-up study had several objectives. Firstly, we wished to identify patients' risk factors which were deemed to cause the initial attack. Secondly, we hoped to identify the factors during first admission which presaged future illness and mortality, and in the case of mortality, the exact mode of death. Thirdly, we looked at aspects of rehabilitation, including the length of stay in hospital following the initial attack, the safety of exercise and the feasibility of returning to work (irrespective of its nature), and to normal driving and to sexual intercourse. (The conservative and restrictive approach to treating coronary patients in the past included prolonged hospitalisation and bed rest, and later prolonged restrictions on exercise, driving, returning to work and sexual intercourse.) Fourthly, we were concerned with establishing the influence of risk factor modification – such as stopping smoking or treating high blood pressure – on subsequent health events, and particularly on mortality from coronary and other causes.

During the early years of the study most patients were followed-up in the hospital or private clinics. In later years, after my retirement in 1988 and Noel Hickey's untimely death in 1994, follow up was by letter or telephone to the patient, their family or family doctor, or by inspecting hospital records and death certificates. Occasionally we depended on a friendly police sergeant to suss out the whereabouts of a non-responder or a particularly reclusive or recalcitrant patient. Not all patients were willing to return to our clinic; and in such cases Noel or I would take to the road and visit patients in various part of the country and once or twice in England. These were far from being disagreeable experiences. Apart from enjoying a visit to the countryside during the summer weekends, we were warmly received by the patients and their families, and we were invariably invited to partake of the 'priest's bottle' at the end of the interview.

Ireland, at least in those years, proved to be an ideal country for such a long-term follow-up study because, unlike many other Western countries, there was little population mobility in town and country and in general we were dealing with an educated society. Only ten lived in England or abroad. Few patients were lost to follow-up, communication was not difficult and English was spoken by all. It is likely that our follow-up study of more than forty years is probably the longest reported case history study into heart disease in the world.

We identified the factors on admission which presaged an adverse long-term prognosis. The most striking result of intervention relating to long-term mortality was the effect of smoking cessation. Among those who were smokers at the time of their first attack, those who stopped had 36 percent mortality after seventeen years, while those who continued to smoke had an 82 percent mortality. We published this report in the *British Heart Journal* and it was the first such finding about the benefits of stopping smoking after a heart attack reported in the medical literature, a first which we shared with a similar report from Gothenburg in Sweden.

We studied the effects of other treatment interventions, including blood pressure and cholesterol control. We found that good blood pressure control was beneficial in terms of mortality, but in these early days we had no effective means of treating high cholesterol levels. However, recent trials elsewhere have convincingly shown that the modern statins drugs improve the prognosis of patients with cholesterol problems.

We advocated a graduated and safe aerobic exercise programme for our patients on discharge from hospital which proved of obvious benefit in terms of increasing their confidence and quality of life. This was a particular challenge to us to ensure that patients continued the programme permanently. Walking was the preferred form of exercise and patients were encouraged to walk up to twenty-one miles a week as an optimum objective.

Not all were so energetic but graduated exercise was of importance in ameliorating or eliminating later angina, particularly when done in conjunction with appropriate risk factor modification and the use of anti-anginal drugs. Like dedicated runners, many patients became addicted to walking and these patients in particular could be relied upon to comply with other lifestyle imperatives. The walkers got a psychological boost and a renewed confidence in returning to a normal life, strengthened by their disciplined adherence to other desirable lifestyle recommendations.

During the initial illness, patients in the wards were encouraged to do regular bed exercises supervised by the twice-daily visit of a physiotherapist with her recorder and suitable musical accompaniment. Unlike the prolonged bed rest of the past, early movement was the rule immediately after the patient's symptoms had subsided. There is little doubt that prolonged bed rest is associated with significant clotting and respiratory complications, which only add to patients' problems in hospital. In a register of data kept in our in-patient service, it is notable that in 1980 an initial average bed stay was about eight days for patients admitted with heart attacks, which had fallen considerably since the 1960s, and had fallen further to six days by 1990. In my earlier days in medicine such patients were hospitalised for six weeks or more. Other major limitations imposed on patients in the past were soon to be dispensed with when it became clear that they involved no special risk.

However, we were aware of the problems which beset the long-term success of achieving lifestyle changes. They included compliance to regular aerobic exercise, stopping and staying off smoking, eating sensibly and taking medications when required. Many patients, despite their best intentions, were prone to recidivism and thus needed constant reinforcement during follow up. We were only too well-aware that the sense of urgency might be lacking in the heart patient who might think that he or she was fully recovered, forgetting that the underlying disease was still lurking below the surface.

In 1971, we reported in the *Journal of the Irish Medical Association* that 93 percent of our patients had returned to their normal work by the end of six months. (Only two patients were advised to change their occupations.) A comparative study of returning to work among male coronary patients in the general population of the same age group as our patients, provided by the Irish Department of Social Security, confirmed a final 40 percent returning to work because of the conservative policies of the profession at the time. It was to take many more years before the profession changed its ways in terms of encouraging an early return to normal life after a heart attack. Among the few who failed to return to work, the reasons were more often social or psychological rather than medical.

Valuable information on the influence of psychological, social and educational factors was collected by the follow-up team of nurses, dietician, psychologist, social worker and physiotherapist. Aspects of compliance to lifestyle changes and on motivation to undertake such changes were also noted. The better-educated were more compliant.

We know from a variety of research studies that the progress of atherosclerosis in the coronary arteries can be retarded and even reversed by methods such as the normalisation of blood cholesterol, the adoption of aerobic exercise programmes, smoking cessation and the use of modern drugs to control cholesterol abnormalities. Controlling the disease in the arteries should be the bedrock of treatment, but has been for many years neglected by the profession in favour of less effective drugs and invasive treatments. The strict application of preventive measures would greatly reduce the need for coronary artery surgery and angioplasty.

Doctors from the beginning of history have been concerned with the treatment of the sick and disabled. Although Hippocrates may have spoken about the maintenance of health as he did about the treatment of the sick (he said 'exercise is the best medicine'), health promotion and prevention has played little part in the medical world during the last two millennia. This tradition is understandable because we are trained to diagnose and treat the sick. We get little or no training in counselling, the bedrock of successful prevention. Many have little insight into the problems of long-term compliance and are committed to the skills they are trained to use rather than providing the lengthy, face-to-face counselling that requires patience and much more time than writing prescriptions or arranging tests. Any general practitioner or cardiologist who sees thirty patients in a session is not practising holistic medicine.

For the ill patient, abreaction in the nature of a quick fix is more likely to alleviate anxiety, even if the remedy is simply a placebo. But, with adequate counselling by the doctor, through explanation and reassurance, the quick fix may not be the answer in terms of real patient benefit. During the last few years, as the profession has tardily accepted the need for rehabilitation of patients recovering from a heart attack, the responsibility to provide these essential services is now largely left to nurses, nutritionists, social workers and other personnel trained in counselling and health promotion. The full multi-trained rehabilitation team has proven to be highly effective and each member of the team learns to deal in a comprehensive way with all patient queries, apart from strictly cardiac issues. In terms of patient confidence and adhesion to long-term advice, these can be enhanced by the interest and participation of the cardiologist. In our service, one of the essential features was the presence of a cardiologist familiar with their medical condition who might be asked to see the patient to advise about their progress and to allay their anxieties.

In the early 1970s I became an actively involved member of the working groups on epidemiology and prevention, and of the working groups of rehabilitation, of the European Society of Cardiology and the International Society and Federation of Cardiology. My adoption of the role of medical epidemiologist was a hugely important addition to my career – I call it an epiphany. Having a busy life as a clinician and at the same time becoming an active epidemiologist should not be a cause for wonder; and yet such a conjunction is rare in our profession. During twenty-five years with my international colleagues, I was one of the very few to have a full clinical appointment in a hospital. Most of our colleagues were in academic positions in universities or hospitals and had no contact with patients. I was probably unique because I added a third aspect to my career in pursuing an active public campaign on the prevention of heart disease. Over the years my secretary collected seven well-filled scrap books which testify to my many public pronouncements on health and lifestyle.

Other research projects included the design of a computerised coronary care register in 1980 designed by Ian Graham. Thus we were provided with information of medical, demographic, social and administrative interest about our in-patients and with information about the changing pattern of disease over time.

Patients in hospital are, as expected, at high risk of sudden death, mostly from sudden heart attacks. We needed to recognise those who were at high risk in order to prevent or treat such an event. As part of his remit, Ian Graham with my registrar, Coleman Ryan (now a cardiologist in San Francisco), carried out a detailed analysis of all cardio-respiratory arrests which occurred in the hospital, all of whom received immediate attention from the ever-vigilant resuscitation team. The object of the survey was to recognise the prodromal features of the high risk cases and record the outcome of resuscitation in different types of clinical circumstances.

One hundred and forty successive arrests occurred in the hospital over a period of fourteen months (about forty arrests occurred in the same patient) and were attended by the resuscitation team on duty. It was possible from the results obtained to predict the type of patient who was likely to recover and those who would not respond to resuscitation. This allowed us to identify the high risk patient who might be kept on the resuscitation list. Most of the patients were not suitable for resuscitation but a clearly defined minority were likely to recover if dealt with promptly. This research work was subsequently published.

Between 1950 and my retirement from medical research in 1992, more than two hundred papers were published by me and my colleagues in peer-reviewed journals, only some of which are included in my *Festshrift*. The full list is in my archives at home. Financial support for our cardiac research at St Vincent's and at the Coombe Lying-in Hospital came from the New Ireland Assurance, Shell and BP, the Department of Health through Ministers Seán McEntee and Charles Haughey, businessmen Patrick Gallagher, Larry Goodman, John Corcoran and a group led by Martin Winston, the British Heart Foundation, the Leverhulme Trust and the European Union.

THE FUTURE OF CARDIOLOGY

What of the future in cardiology? There may be further advances in diagnostic and therapeutic areas but it is likely that, if past experience is any guide, these will evolve with diminishing cost-effectiveness, at least in the context of the public health and of increasing longevity. It may be possible to dispense with the heart/lung machine for coronary artery surgery or indeed to dispense with coronary surgery in its current form because of improving medical treatment or new, less invasive techniques.

Intra-luminal intervention through angioplasty may be further improved in its effectiveness although it urgently needs to be more fully validated.

Because of the paucity of donor hearts, heart transplants will never be easily available and must be confined to the rare patient who is in the right place at the right time. There will almost certainly be a breakthrough in the development of a mechanical or electronic heart or in the replacement of heart muscle through genetic engineering. However, whether such means of replacing a functioning heart will benefit humanity is in doubt. The artificial heart may lead to further prolongation of life and the loss of a good quality of life and of independence – the living death of Ivan Illich.

Those who are prone to the rare non-coronary causes of sudden death may be identified at an early stage and may be the subject of prophylactic control. This rare but tragic problem in young people is currently being investigated by my son, David, in Tallaght Hospital. Better control of heart irregularities can be envisioned through invasive or remote techniques of ablation or radio transmission. We may find the cause or causes of the rare heart muscle diseases, the cardiomyopathies; and the treatment of heart failure, whatever its cause, may continue to improve.

We shall undoubtedly continue to improve the imaging of the heart and arteries to the point of visualising every structure and function of the organ; but whether this facility will improve our capacity to benefit the patient remains to be seen. Imaging techniques may lead to increasing methods of treatment through non-invasive means. We shall learn more about the mechanisms of clotting and atherosclerosis through cellular research and other basic research methods. Progress in these areas will serve to improve our approach, both in terms of prevention and treatment. It is in more fully understanding the causes and mechanisms of atherosclerosis and its complications that holds the only promise of achieving a final conquest over the twentieth-century epidemic of coronary heart disease.

Heart disease will lose its current dominance as one of the major contributors to illness in our society. Coronary disease may eventually be simply a distant memory. We may improve the health of the community, even beyond our current hopes, but the cost of our health services will continue to rise with more expensive and sophisticated investigations and management techniques, and as we become more efficient at keeping the very old and infirm alive, which itself involves serious ethical and practical problems.

As a latter-day Luddite, I question the benefits of our incessant search for the means of postponing the inevitability of death and to challenge our natural surroundings. As the Angel Rafael said to Adam (according to John Milton in *Paradise Lost*) 'Do not try to understand the stars.' There are other and greater challenges to be faced. The degradation of the planet, the plundering of nature and the burgeoning world population may make the future of cardiology irrelevant.

9

INTERNATIONAL RESEARCH INTO CORONARY DISEASE

My first contact with international rehabilitation workers was at the World Congress of Cardiology in London in 1971. The members were mostly active cardiologists with ambitions to improve the management of patients who were recovering from heart attacks. They came from many European countries, including from Eastern Europe. We had not yet met with the American rehabilitation group. The Europeans were obviously a progressive group but at the time of my meeting with them they were still strongly influenced by the more conservative and cautious approach which prevailed in the management of heart attack patients during the acute stage and during convalescence. We presented a paper at the rehabilitation section of the congress which reported results in our male patients younger than sixty who survived a first heart attack and who were encouraged to take up aerobic exercise, to follow advice about risk factors and to return to work at an earlier date. Their duration of hospitalisation was short compared to the traditional custom of many of my colleagues at the congress.

Our findings were in striking contrast to the traditional approach to such patients who were hospitalised for many weeks and were subjected to strict bed rest. Many of these restrictive ·recommendations were still in vogue in 1970, particularly in delaying a return to work and following a prolonged convalescence. Our results – 75 percent of patients returning to work after three months, 93 percent after six months and only two patients, both drivers of passenger vehicles, changing jobs – were received with some degree of incredulity by our British and European colleagues. From 1970 I became closely involved with this European rehabilitation group. Henri Denolin of Brussels led the working party in our early years, a father figure whose leadership was an inspiration to us all. And later, in 1979, a formal working group of the European Society of Cardiology (ESC) was formed under the joint chairmanship of Peter Mathes of Höhenried, Germany and myself. I remained as co-chairman until my retirement from international activities in 1992.

The European approach to cardiac rehabilitation which I encountered was influenced by the German spa tradition. It was more formal and less effective than ours. After a somewhat prolonged stay in hospital, patients were returned home for about two months' convalescence before return-ing as out-patients or going to a special rehabilitation hospital or spa for a formal programme of callisthenic exercise under the supervision of a spe-cially-trained physiotherapist and for assessment by a psychologist and appropriate counselling. At that time the approach by the members of the group was mainly concerned with exercise and stress. Stress and personal-ity type were for a long time considered important in the United States as well as Europe in causing a susceptibility to coronary disease but have since received little attention.

The institutional programme continued for about four weeks, at which point the patient was returned home to the care of his or her family practitioner. There was no emphasis on risk factor identification and intervention, and the long-term need for adherence to an exercise regime was neglected despite the proven necessity of constant reinforcement for patients to make permanent changes in lifestyle.

Despite our report to the group in London in 1970, the Europeans were slow to adopt our more practical and sensible clinical approach to rehabilitation. The traditional European practices continued for many years, particularly in the central and eastern European countries. The British were almost unique in that they had apparently no interest in rehabilitation although Elizabeth Cay of Edinburgh, Scotland was a good contributor. The British were largely influenced by the Hammersmith Hospital cardiologists who were the leaders in interventionist cardiology.

In our earlier research into causes of heart disease we employed a psychologist but we were unable to link coronary disease with any psychological or personality factors, although stress is difficult to define and more difficult to measure. Anxiety and mood changes, which are largely related to the patient's illness, are likely to be best managed by the cardiologist rather than a clinically more remote psychologist. Internationally, stress and personality type eventually was no longer believed as increasing a propensity to coronary disease.

For the next twenty years I visited almost every major country in Europe as a member of the European rehabilitation working party, often accompanied by my colleague Noel Hickey. Our system of rehabilitation, which was simply based on good clinical practice, continued to be different from the more academic approach of the Europeans during most of my active clinical days. It was not until 1980, when the Irish Heart Foundation organised a joint meeting in Dublin of the rehabilitation and the epidemiology and prevention working groups of the European Society, that risk factor identification and intervention was gradually added to the policies of our European colleagues.

Because the European approach to rehabilitation remained along more formal and institutional lines, our different policies within the group led to some rather unusual situations. A cardiac rehabilitation meeting of the World Health Organisation was organised in Prague in 1975. On our way to Prague Noel Hickey and I decided to fly to Vienna and to travel the short distance to our destination by train. However, this was during the Cold War and we found to our consternation that there was no means of crossing the frontier between Vienna and Prague. After hectic enquiries we found that we could go to Brno in Slovakia by train, which we did that evening. At Brno a friendly officer who seemed anxious to practise his English, slipped us into the officers' compartment of a troop train which was fortuitously going to Prague that night. During the journey we were interviewed by an inspector on a few occasions; we were told, not to leave the train, but to move to the coaches where the soldiers were packed like sardines. We did not understand the various languages he employed and our loyal officer friend refused to translate by pretending that he had no English. We continued in the relative luxury of our coach and arrived in Prague the next morning late and exhausted, but grateful to our Good Samaritan.

The meeting was dominated by the members of the European working party who favoured the traditional formal rehabilitation approach. After a few days' discussion it was decided to set up a research programme to test the value of rehabilitation. The protocol of the enquiry was to be prepared and referred to another meeting in Moscow about six months later. It was to be based on the groups' formal European approach, that is, time in hospital (phase 1); recovery period at home for two months (phase 2); admission to rehabilitation institute for one month's exercise training and for nutritional and psychological advice (phase 3) and return home under the care of a family doctor or local cardiologist (phase 4). At the end of the meeting the chairman went around the table to ascertain who would be willing to go to Moscow to participate in the research. All agreed to do so but when he questioned Noel and myself, we were obliged to answer that we could not participate because most of our patients would be back at work before phase 3. Nevertheless, the WHO chairman insisted that we should attend in an advisory capacity, which indeed we were glad to do and so I had my first visit to Moscow.

Noel and I went to Moscow as planned six months later. We joined in the discussions on the research project but we had little hope that it would lead to useful results. The system adopted was too impractical for clinical practice and there was widespread lack of suitable phase 3 rehabilitation institutions. Germany might have been one country which could have provided such institutions because, after the war, the country was left with a large number of spas which were no longer included in their health service. Perhaps the best-known rehabilitation centre in Germany was in Höhenried, outside Munich. The head of the institute, Max Halhuber, was warm, sociable and larger than life; he and his wife, who was also a doctor and involved in rehabilitation, were excellent hosts. He was devoted to the old German spa tradition and these outdated institutions made excellent rehabilitation centres in terms of the traditional European approach. From 1976 onwards it was a feature of several of our meetings in Europe that Halhuber and I would give a joint talk entitled 'Protagonist and Antagonist' where we would each present the merits of our different systems of rehabilitation and what we perceived to be the drawbacks of our opponent's approach. He would always finish his address with the intended compliment that I did not need their formal institutional system as I was myself an institution!

My travels around Europe as a member of the rehabilitation and epidemiology working parties of the ESC led to many meetings and to a number of enduring friendships. But I often wonder whether these repeated meetings led to the better clinical treatment of heart patients at the international level. It was not easy for a small, committed group, restricted to a specialist area of medicine which had no great appeal to many of our more invasive and drug-committed clinical colleagues, to communicate its views to the profession and to the public at large. However, we probably did influence the various heart foundations in Europe, and through them the public. There was, however, a sense of futility and doubt at times of speaking only to the converted, as we met so often and there seemed to be little variation in our discussions. Even in 2010, the medical journals are still regurgitating the same papers that we were publishing thirty years ago.

We celebrated the twentieth anniversary of the foundation of our rehabilitation working party in Munich in 2004. It was hosted by Peter Mathes, who had been my co-chairman until I retired in 1992 and had also succeeded Max Halhuber as director of the Höhenried Rehabilitation Institute. It was fortuitous that I was able to report the Irish initiative to ban smoking in public places, which had just been adopted that year, thanks to pressure from the Irish Heart Foundation, the Irish Cancer Society and Irish Ash, and the unprecedented response of Mícheál Martin, our then-minister for health. My European friends were duly impressed and full of enquiries about the circumstances and strategies which led to such a successful outcome. I believe myself that the biggest factor influencing the government was the threat of litigation by the bar staff exposed to secondary inhalation of tobacco smoke in the public houses and hotels.

I joined the rehabilitation working group of the International Society and Federation of Cardiology (IFSC) during the 1970s, which was chaired by Nanette Wenger of Atlanta, Georgia in the United States. Nanette was an energetic and dynamic chairperson and an outstanding organiser. She dominated her international colleagues during my entire membership of the group. Her leadership and writings have made a major contribution to the management of coronary patients. This group had a more realistic approach to the long-term management of coronary patients. We met every year in various parts of the world and our group undoubtedly played an important role in advancing the more practical and effective management of coronary patients. I and my research staff contributed to the international literature that was published by the group, mostly organised by Nanette Wenger.

I was a founder member of the IFSC working group on epidemiology established after the World Congress in 1971. It was the major source of activity in relation to the study of heart disease in populations, both in terms of training epidemiologists and in inspiring research into the population trends and causes of coronary disease, stroke and high blood pressure. It was up-to-date with the many studies that were taking place worldwide and it undertook important international collaborative studies in relation to nutrition, salt, and high blood pressure. Although I was a constant attendee at the meetings of the working group, I did not take part in any of its major population studies because of my clinical and research responsibilities at home and my need to make a living through private practice. However, the meetings and my close contact with the world's leading epidemiologists and medical statisticians had a profound influence on my career in medicine and particularly in the design and organisation of our own follow-up study of young coronary patients. The IFSC working group was led by some of the most prominent epidemiologists, mostly from English-speaking and Scandinavian countries, and was to have a profound influence on the control of the cardiovascular diseases in the western world.

A highlight every year was the ten-day teaching session which was organised by the IFSC epidemiology working group. These sessions were designed to educate young medical graduates (and sometimes the not-so-young) to enter the ranks of medical epidemiology. They were hugely popular and unfortunately each ten-day event was limited to about twenty pupils. They were held in different countries throughout the world; they were residential and usually held in some out-of-the way place. The intimacy of these training sessions led to many lasting friendships, to the formation of close networks of communication in the field of medical epidemiology and to the spreading of the techniques and the organisation of population research worldwide. The IFSC working group made a seminal contribution to the control of the coronary epidemic.

The annual training session was the brain child of Jeremiah Stamler of Chicago and his wife Rose. Rose, sadly, died a few years ago, but Jerry lived to celebrate his ninetieth birthday last January, a splendid example of heeding his own advice. The teaching faculty was made up of our leading members, including the Stamlers, Geoffrey Rose, Henry Blackburn, and a scattering of other experts from around the world. The faculty was supported by a leading medical statistician who was by nature demanding and despotic, and control of the organisation was in the capable hands of Rose Stamler. I did not have the opportunity to join the faculty because of my clinical commitments, nor was I qualified to take a teaching role. However I did attend the second of these teaching sessions, which was held in Byrne's Hotel (recently sold to developers) in Blessington, County Wicklow, then a sleepy country village; it was sponsored by the Irish Heart Foundation. The faculty as well as students, despite a heavy teaching programme, learned the virtues of Guinness as a restorative and generator of good conversation. Blessington is now part of our rural sprawl and the commuter belt, and is no longer a suitable location for such intimate academic groups. On our two half days devoted to recreation, we paid visits to the monastic site in Glendalough and to Newgrange and the ancient relics on the Boyne. They were a source of interest and wonder to those visiting us from afar.

In my meetings with various organisations, I met all the outstanding figures in the rehabilitation world and in cardiovascular epidemiology and took part in many working party meetings and larger congresses. I was a member of various advisory groups about heart disease prevention and rehabilitation, including the WHO, the European Community, the British Cardiac Society and our own government. As well as enjoying the academic aspects of the working groups, I had good reasons to enjoy the social part of the meetings and the company and friendship of kindred spirits.

I paid my second visit to Moscow to attend the World Congress of Cardiology. On our arrival we were immediately entertained by the

Ministry of Health at a drinks party, which was hosted by the minister. At one stage I was sipping a small glass of vodka when the minister himself came over to me and said, in guttural English, 'You must not drink vodka that way. You must throw it back. Otherwise you will get drunk!'

Restaurants were apparently few and it was virtually impossible to book a table. However, on the night of our arrival our leader from the ministry brought us to a restaurant, outside of which there was a queue of at least thirty people waiting. As we arrived at the back of the queue he lifted a document in his hand and shouted, 'We are the guests of the Ministry of Health!' and promptly the crowd divided meekly to let us through.

One day I was running along the Moscow River when I met two other runners, who were American; otherwise during my two visits to that city I saw no others running. In questioning one of my Russian hosts later, I asked why the Muscovites did not run. He replied with great authority that it had once been fashionable in Russia, but that they soon discovered that running was dangerous and was best avoided! He may have been right, for I never encountered such hard concrete as that along the Moscow River! These were still the days of communism, and I found some of my Russian colleagues to be very dismissive of Western – or rather, American – culture. The hotel I stayed in during my first visit, the Rossi, was newly built. It was a huge block with 1,500 bedrooms, run like an army camp, with a formidable female commissar in charge of each floor; she was called a *babushka*, the Russian for 'grandmother'. Residents were obliged to report to their floor's *babushka* on arriving and leaving their room.

Moscow had some merit: it had the Kremlin with its vast museum, a few beautiful churches with their icons, their ornate exteriors and their multicoloured bulbous 'onion domes' so evocative of the East, and the Pushkin Gallery, with its magnificent collection of Impressionist paintings.

I visited East Berlin, with its wall still intact, on my way home. It, on the other hand, appeared to have no merit. The hotel was modern-American in style but more banana-republic in function and facilities. East Berlin was a newly rebuilt concrete desert, with vast box-like apartment blocks lining wide boulevards with little traffic; the shops seemed empty of consumer goods. Compensation for me was provided by my daily five-kilometre run from the hotel to the infamous Checkpoint Charlie and back. It was to me the great landmark and symbol of the Cold War. Imagine my surprise when, on my arrival at the checkpoint, I found a small, inconspicuous door in the great wall guarded by a single soldier carrying a rifle. No tanks, no machine-guns, no barbed wire and none of the outdoor furniture one might expect to service a battalion of men dedicated to controlling a discontented citizenry.

I must, however, acknowledge the kindness of my colleagues in East Berlin, Professor Heiner Gunther. Although the East German looked askance at my addiction to running, they provided me with the warmest hospitality under difficult circumstances. My host was the head of a large hospital, the Charité. It was widely believed that he was high in the ranks of the Communist Party and I am told that he was sacked after the wall came down. His prominence in the Party seemed likely, as we were treated as VIPs on the plane from Moscow; all were held back while we boarded from a VIP lounge. We were seated in front and passengers were not permitted to stand up in the plane on arrival in Berlin until we were lead to the rear entrance, much to the protest of a few American passengers. Even the cult of communism was impervious to the temptations of power and personal privilege.

10

HIGH BLOOD PRESSURE (HYPERTENSION)

Blood pressure was first measured by the Rev. Stephen Hales in 1773 by inserting the end of a long glass column full of water into the artery of a horse. He found that the column of blood which rushed out reaching over eight feet in height. Today, we use the sphygmomanometer, a cuff around the upper arm which, when inflated can identify the systolic and diastolic pressure levels by characteristic sounds heard by a stethoscope held over the artery below the cuff. It was first invented by Riva Rocci in 1896. We use a vertical glass tube containing mercury, which is fourteen times denser than water, to record the pressures in millimetres of mercury. Digital instruments are more compact than the original sphygmo-manometer and are also widely available. The arbitrary figures of 120/80 hg mm (millimetres of mercury) are accepted as normal, but there are wide variations of normality around this figure. The blood pressure some-times changes in the body in response to various physical and emotional circumstances; it tends to remain steady and at a relatively low level while at rest in bed.

Normal blood pressure should not increase with age, except for a slight rise and a greater lability in systolic pressure caused by the arteries becoming more rigid in older people and their more sluggish reflexes controlling blood pressure on standing. Because of wide daytime variations in blood pressure, particularly as we grow older, it is important that we should never make a diagnosis of high blood pressure based on only one or two readings. Patients under stress may have a transient rise in blood pressure, often described as the 'white coat effect' when consulting a doctor. Before confirming a diagnosis, a twenty-four-hour continuous blood pressure recording should be arranged. It is not easy to say when the blood pressure is abnormally raised, but any persistent level above 150/90 should be investigated, particularly in younger people. Such a level would certainly call for appropriate lifestyle changes and might require a blood pressure reducing drug.

After the prevention and treatment of coronary heart disease, essential hypertension, the most common type formed the next most important part of my practice and research. High blood pressure caused by kidney disease was common sixty years ago but gradually became a relative rarity following the introduction of penicillin in the late 1940s. It was the common basis of malignant hypertension, so called because it proceeded inexorably to fatal stroke, heart failure or kidney failure. Essential hypertension, almost certainly a lifestyle condition and still common today, has a more benign natural history but, if not controlled, can eventually lead to an accelerated phase and to heart failure, stroke or coronary disease. It was only in later years that we identified high blood pressure as an important determinant of coronary disease, particularly in communities prone to high blood cholesterol.

Unlike hypertension stemming from kidney disease, essential hypertension is eminently treatable by appropriate lifestyle changes and by the plethora of effective drugs which are now on the market. High blood pressure should therefore cease to be a major problem in clinical practice, but unfortunately it is not always adequately treated, nor are patients always compliant with treatment advice.

It is essential that the severity and lability of the patient's blood pressure is identified before medication is commenced. There is little need to begin immediate treatment with drugs except in the rare case when severe high blood pressure and associated significant symptoms come to one's notice for the first time. In many non-urgent cases, it is possible to avoid medication by non-pharmacological methods, including exercise programmes, control of obesity, salt and alcohol limitation, and the reduction of chronic stress.

Drug treatment requires careful dosage review over a period of time once high blood pressure has been established. The twenty-four-hour monitor, which has reached a high standard of accuracy and reliability, can provide serial readings and it has greatly advanced our knowledge of the natural history of blood pressure. With appropriate treatment, it should be possible to keep blood pressure at normal or close-to-normal levels. Inadequate drug treatment can result from excessive caution on the part of the doctor or poor adherence to the prescription by the patient. Excessive treatment will lead to side-effects where the blood pressure drops excessively, causing dizziness or fainting, particularly when standing from the sitting or lying positions.

The wide variety of drugs which are effective in controlling blood pressure should provide an opportunity to find a suitable medication without side-effects. The most universal failure among patients and the profession has been the neglect of the lifestyle aspects of blood pressure control. In my experience, patients who have confirmed essential hypertension are often able to dispense with the use of drugs if appropriate lifestyle changes are made. Medication can be resumed if there is a tendency for the pressure to increase.

With initial training by the nurse or doctor, regular self-monitoring of blood pressure can be effectively taught to and managed by the great majority of patients. It involves the patient and his or her family in blood pressure management, a situation which greatly improves patient compliance to long-term treatment and which goes a long way towards helping the patient stay on the correct medication and adhere to recommended lifestyle habits.

The epidemiology of high blood pressure has been the subject of a considerable amount of research. We have strong epidemiological evidence that it is a lifestyle-induced disease – that is, it strongly points to 'nurture' rather than 'nature' being at its roots (although it is possible that there may be genetically-vulnerable individuals). Research confirms that high blood pressure is related to the salt intake of populations: it is a common condition in Western countries and is rare in many African and

Asian countries, particularly in primitive communities where salt intake is very low. Essential hypertension complicated by cerebral haemorrhage or heart failure has been a major cause of death in Japan, at least until recent times, and this could be attributed to the very high salt content of the Japanese diet. It is less common among Japanese who emigrate to other countries, where their dietary pattern may change and conform more to that of their host country. In the United States, high blood pressure and its complications are more prevalent in African-Americans than in American Caucasians, almost certainly because the African-Americans came from places where salt intake was traditionally extremely low. An adverse response to salt is thus likely to be greater than among Caucasians who originate mostly from Europe, where salt intake has always been high, even as far back as Roman times.

There is also strong epidemiological evidence that the people in countries with a high salt intake are prone to developing cancer of the stomach. The recent dramatic fall in stomach cancer in Western countries may be partly or largely attributed to the decline in salt intake and the refrigeration of food during the last half century. There is little doubt that limitation of salt in a population will contribute to a better life expectancy. The early fall in stroke mortality which was evident by the 1950s in Western countries can be attributed largely to the control of kidney disease, but the continued fall in recent years owes itself to the increasing use of blood pressure medication, to food preservation by refrigeration, to reduced intake of salt at the table and reduced salt usage by the food industries. In former times, much salt was used in food preservation, and those of us who lived in the earlier part of the twentieth century will recall the barrels and containers of salt used to preserve fish and other foods. We will also recall the liberal use of free salt at the table. I appeared on *The Late Late Show* about thirty years ago on the subject of salt, blood pressure and heart disease, and I believe, from the reaction of the public and the salt industry who commented about the programme, that my appearance had some influence on salt consumption in Ireland.

11

EVIDENCE, DRUGS AND PREVENTION

IS MEDICINE EVIDENCE-BASED?

As a clinical cardiologist with a considerable commitment to prevention and to unnecessary interventions, I have always thought that there was too much surgery advocated for the treatment of patients with coronary disease. Medical and surgical interventions up to the mid-twentieth century were based on traditional empirical grounds and had little scientific or experimental basis to justify them. In retrospect, many of these treatment methods were valueless and not infrequently harmful to the patient. In recent years, there has been an increasing interest in and commitment to evidence-based medicine by the profession in terms of clinical trials and population studies by epidemiologists. Despite our latter-day commitment to proper trials, many aspects of medical treatment, including in my own speciality of cardiology, are still based on poor or no evidence. Examples are the inappropriate use of drugs and the overuse of coronary surgery and angioplasty. They have never been properly evaluated, and some forms of treatment are practised despite well-established basic and clinical research which throws serious doubt on their efficacy. Too often our commitment to evidence-based medicine is more a vague aspiration rather than based on real evidence. Claude Bernard, the great French physiologist, in his introduction to *The Study of Experimental Medicine*, published in 1855, wrote,

> A physician who tries a remedy and cures his patient is inclined to believe that the cure is due to his treatment. But the first thing to ask them is if they tried doing nothing, that is, not treating other patients, for how can they otherwise know whether the remedy or nature cured them?

Was this the first plea for evidence-based medicine? At its best, the practice of medicine is an amalgam of prevention and treatment. That doctors are a conservative lot is evident in many areas of medicine. That is, except when some new drug or intervention is introduced with acclamation and which may be widely prescribed, often before its efficacy has been properly confirmed by appropriate clinical trials. Hence the litany of drugs which have been widely prescribed for heart disease in recent years, and which ultimately were found to be useless or even harmful.

In a paper we published in 1981 in the *American Journal of Cardiology*, we described the outcome in terms of complications and mortality in a hundred successive males who were admitted under our care with a diagnosis of heart attack, called 'unstable angina'. We used none of the drugs which were in vogue at the time and which were then almost routinely used in international practice. These included drugs such as beta-blockers and calcium blockers, among others. Our policy was to encourage immediate life-style change and an early return to normal life. Despite many other reports of unstable angina where 'intensive medical treatment' was employed with a variety of drugs, we concluded by writing that current drug treatment requires confirmation and:

> Our own experience suggests that a conservative approach to treatment within the coronary care unit, using drugs only when symptomatically indicated, may be equally effective.

In other words, the drugs in fashion may be of no value. This paper received editorial comment, including:

> Although their study may not effect a major change in the direction of present management of patients with unstable angina pectoris, the results dispel complacency relative to complete satisfaction with current management of such patients in the United States.

Our contribution had little or no effect on the profession, nor am I aware of any other centre deciding to emulate our experiment.

During my first twenty years as consultant cardiologist at St Vincent's Hospital I submitted about 150 patients with mitral stenosis to surgery. The results of the operation were good and, as one finds in many other operations, as the learning curve reached its apogee, mortality and complication rates following surgery became quite infrequent. It was natural to attribute the improved health and greater longevity of our patients to the operation but there were other confounding factors which may have added to our good results.

The disease was most common among the poor and destitute. From the time of the Second World War, the conditions in the poorer sections of the community in Dublin began to improve. Infections, malnutrition, anaemia and exposure all contributed to deterioration and early death in patients with rheumatic heart disease. Better housing, improved nutrition and better clothing, combined with advances in our medical services, dramatically improved the lot of the poor. After the war, patients attending specialised cardiac services, such as mine at St Vincent's Hospital and the Coombe Lying-in Hospital, were protected from the worst effects of poor social conditions by virtue of general medical supervision and care. Hence it is difficult to assess the quantitative effect surgery had on long-term improved health and longevity because of these and other possible confounding factors.

To confirm the true value of surgery, we would have needed a properly designed trial where an adequate number of patients with mitral stenosis would be operated on and a similar number of carefully matched patients would be treated by conservative means. These patients would be chosen randomly to eliminate bias in allotting them to each category. This is the model of the proper randomised trial but, in the case of the treatment of mitral disease, you can be certain that such a trial has never been held because the rationale of surgery would make it difficult to deny our patients the apparent benefits of the operation. Hence, we cannot be certain what benefit, if any, we were conferring on our mitral patients by subjecting them to surgery.

It is not always easy to design and execute a randomised control trial in medicine and sometimes providing comparable enough patients and controls can prove impossible. Too many trials are badly designed or subject to bias, thus raising considerable doubt about some of our treatment methods. A research team requires considerable experience, including expert statistical advice, in designing, executing and interpreting medical trials of drug and surgical interventions.

The same dilemma was to occur many years later after the advent of coronary surgery at the end of the 1970s when patients with coronary heart disease were offered heart surgery as a first measure. About the same time we saw the slow but gradual adoption of appropriate lifestyle changes by patients aimed at the reduction or regression of the underlying coronary artery disease and, more recently, effective drugs. In the case of coronary heart disease and in the absence of proper trials, it is equally difficult to quantify the part surgery plays in benefiting the patient when adequate secondary prevention is achieved through appropriate lifestyle changes and appropriate drug therapy. Too many unnecessary heart operations were and are being performed. Many coronary patients submitted to heart surgery will do at least as well or better in terms of avoiding further symptoms or complications and in terms of longevity, and can avoid the not-inconsiderable added complications of expense and the inconvenience of invasive interventions.

It is ironic that, despite our growing commitment to evidence-based medicine, much treatment of heart disease is not supported by reliable trial evidence. I refer in particular to the worldwide adoption of coronary artery surgery and to angioplasty procedures. Early trials of heart surgery indicated the value of the procedure in certain and limited high-risk patients, so that in the 1970s and early 1980s we had a rational basis for surgical intervention in such cases. Because advancement is a continuous process in all areas of medicine, it may be necessary to review the validity of our treatments from time to time in order to ensure that we are prac-tising the best medicine.

Since the early trials of heart surgery there have been dramatic advances in medical treatment which are very often the best alternative approach to surgery and angioplasty. The new approach of angioplasty has made great progress and surgical techniques themselves have advanced considerably. However, while cardiologists have neglected proper medical treatment in the past, they are now gradually accepting that medical treat-ment is crucially important in patients, whether or not they are submitted to surgery. The great advances in medical treatment and surgery, and the introduction of angioplasty, make the original trials irrelevant and there are no satisfactory recent trials now to guide us in the correct treatment of coronary patients. The evidence available from clinical experience where medical treatment is properly prescribed and from international studies of the factors which account for the recent major decline in heart mortality would suggest that too many patients are subjected to heart surgery and to angioplasty. In my long clinical and research experience, and our fol-low-ups of patients for forty years, I have no doubt that these invasive interventions are frequently unjustified.

Angioplasty was adopted worldwide without proper trials. Angioplasty is a procedure where a fine tube or catheter with an inflatable balloon at its tip is introduced into a coronary artery from the leg or arm and, by inflating the balloon, blockages in the artery can be distended to improve blood flow. It was first performed by Andreas Greuntzig of Switzerland in 1977 on a human. He had earlier done some successful research on the procedure on animals and in dealing with leg vessel disease in humans. Angioplasty in the heart and leg arteries is not without its problems of medical complications, not to mention its contribution to cost to the patient and the health service. It is employed in dealing with acute prob-lems as well as chronic conditions such as angina of effort or healthy peo-ple who have been prescribed a 'routine' angiogram and found to have a blockage in a coronary artery. Once introduced, angioplasty was adopted worldwide without any clinical trials to confirm its indications and its benefits over non-surgical medical treatment. It is only recently that one acceptable clinical trial has been reported and the results of this trial are equivocal to say the least and do not support such a procedure in many clearly defined patients on grounds of efficacy, cost and complications. There were some previous trials which were not sufficiently well-designed to guide us and, again, the findings, for what they were worth, did not support the use of angioplasty.

I am not qualified to give an opinion about the use of angioplasty in the acutely ill as has been developed in more recent years – it may well be important and may account for the recent improvement in the treatment of acute heart attacks – but I can say without any doubt that its widespread use in the patient with non-acute problems or who has no symptoms is quite unjustified, at least in terms of lack of proof and of the advances provided by modern medical treatment. There is no evidence that a patient without symptoms who has a routine angiogram which identifies one or more blockages is helped by angioplasty. Yet such patients are frequently subjected to the procedure. Indeed the prescription of a 'routine' angiogram is not justified unless the patient is perceived clinically as a possible candidate for an invasive treatment procedure. The performance of such a 'routine' test raises serious ethical problems and is a reflection of the poor audit standards of the profession.

I have published the evidence to confirm my opinions on these issues. It appeared in the *Irish Medical Journal* in February 2006 but it gave rise to no comment from the medical establishment. The very limited trials which are available show, if anything, that medical treatment is marginally better than angioplasty in the non-acute case and if medical treatment were to include strict risk factor control, angioplasty would become a distinct loser.

The European Society of Cardiology decided about five years ago to investigate the reasons cardiological practice appeared to differ in the various heart centres across Europe. I wrote to the president of the society and to the editor of its publication, the *European Heart Journal*. The theme of my letter was that differences were inevitable if we continued to practice treatments and carry out procedures without adequate trial evidence of efficacy. I received no reply to my comments nor am I aware that my letter was considered by the executive of the ESC or published in its journal. It does seem reasonable that we should ponder the question of variations in practice if we wish to claim that modern medicine is based on scientific principles.

THE CURRENT DRUG CULTURE

While many drugs are effective and often lifesaving, drugs used in clinical practice, particularly when used inappropriately, are a frequent cause of significant side effects. Research worldwide has confirmed that up to 20 percent of all hospital admissions and prolonged hospital stays can be attributed to inappropriate drug management or interactions, to patient sensitivity or intolerance, to other interventions (such as surgery) or complications caused by medical intervention or the use of tests. Such problems are called iatrogenic diseases (Greek *iatros* = healing).

One feature of our practice at St Vincent's during my years was a healthy scepticism about the use of the many drugs which were prescribed for heart patients, both during the acute phase of the illness and convalescence and after recovery. This scepticism earned me and my colleague, Noel Hickey, a reputation of being therapeutic nihilists. John O'Sullivan, who was my registrar in 1971, and my senior house officer, Patrick Leavy, kept a careful note of the drugs that one hundred successive patients were taking at the time of admission to the coronary care unit. Among those who survived their illness, their drugs on discharge were noted. They left hospital taking substantially fewer drugs and, in our estimation, only on medications which were deemed appropriate to their medical condition. Some patients even left hospital without any medications. This must have been unique among cardiologists dealing with coronary patients but our policies were based strictly on acceptable trial evidence, on our insights derived from our epidemiological experience and training, and on appropriate lifestyle advice for each patient. The results of this investigation were published in the *Journal of the Royal College of Physicians* in London in 1989. Similar accounts of inappropriate drug-prescribing are reported widely in the medical literature.

Unfortunately, much routine drug prescribing is part of a culture which is less rigorous in demanding proper trials of their efficacy. As I have said, I can cite numerous examples of drugs being used extensively in cardiological practice which eventually proved to be of no therapeutic value. Their use was based on earlier trials but subsequent (and perhaps more independent) trials and clinical experience proved them to be ineffective and in some cases of having undesirable side-effects. These earlier trials were invariably organised and financed by the drug companies, usually in association with clinical doctors and may have been subject to problems of bias.

In 2007 the bill for the Community Drug Scheme in Ireland was €1.74 billion, a five-fold increase since 1997. Their cost was 13.5 percent of all health spending according to a recent report in the *Irish Medical Journal*; and this figure does not include much over-the-counter spending. The profession has largely failed to keep up with drug technology and this can be attributed to the huge pressure and influence of the drug companies, to the bewildering number of drugs available and to the failure of the medical profession to provide conditions in training and practice to ensure that doctors are competent to practise according to the current pharmacopoeia. We sometimes fail to appreciate the limitations of the individual doctor to master the complexities of the drug situation despite the regular publications of the Irish Medicines Board keeping us up-to-date on the side-effects of medications.

Some of the overuse and inappropriate use of drugs is related to corrupt practices among the pharmaceutical companies in association with some physicians and medical academics. There have been several instances of corruption in the design, interpretation and reporting of trials and such practices are ignored or encouraged in some academic institutions and universities and by the medical journals, many of which are dependent on financial support from the industry. Too many medical institutions are now dependent on the drug industry for financial support and can hardly be expected to question some of the unprofessional and corrupt practices which exist; nor can the editors of medical journals be expected to employ the same strict peer review standards as is done with scientific articles, or to be too critical of drug advertisements upon which their journals largely depend for their existence.

An article titled 'Drug Companies and Doctors: a Story of Corruption', in the *New York Review of Books* of 15 January 2009, refers to many cases of gross corruption arising from conflicts of interests between the pharmaceutical industry, physicians, hospitals and other medical institutions. There are many other references in the above publication to the reported widespread corruption in for-profit hospitals in America because of unnecessary surgery and other unprofessional and unethical medical practices. Even our most academic and prestigious medical institutions, such as our Royal Colleges, are beholden to the drug and instrument companies by accepting financial support for their training and academic activities. I suppose only a perfect world would have no drug advertising, where instead doctors would have access to an updated pharmacopoeia and would be subjected to more stringent peer review.

Poor standards can only be remedied by stricter audit of professional practice and by a system of corporate audit in hospital practice. Ideally, an official and updated formulary would be provided by the HSE, and the pressure of drug industry advertising and promotions would be eliminated. (It is appropriate to note the our own *Irish Medical Journal* is one of the few medical journals which does not include drug advertisements.)

Another factor in the abuse of drugs is the widespread use of 'prophylactics', such as the prescribing of aspirin and statins (cholesterol controlling drugs) in healthy people. It is hardly realistic that healthy people should be put on such routine drugs when adhering to simple lifestyle habits would clearly lead to every prospect of good health and longevity. Yet tens of thousands of people in Ireland, particularly among the elderly, are now taking these drugs permanently and have become dependent psychologically as well as physically on doctors. Doctors should be involved in health promotion but much of recent preventive medicine among general practitioners is based more on using drugs rather than advising about healthy lifestyles. Too many patients with borderline abnormalities, such as a raised blood sugar, cholesterol or blood pressure would be better advised about lifestyle. Borderline problems of this type will respond if the subject adheres to advice. If they do not respond because of poor adherence or for other reasons, then the question of medication should be considered. In my experience, in our current drug culture the great majority of doctors will commence medication before such a more rational approach is adopted.

I suspect a real connection between the overuse of legitimate drugs by the profession and the widespread illicit drug culture which is afflicting human society today. As regards illicit drugs, I have been writing to the popular press and to politicians supporting the recommendations of other writers and correspondents who favour decriminalising all drugs. When John Bruton was president of the European Union in 1996, I suggested that he set up a European commission to examine the feasibility of decriminalising drugs. I greatly admired Bruton's leadership qualities and hoped he might accept the challenge. He had the courtesy to reply at considerable length to my suggestion. His letter included fifteen policy points of action intended to address the drug problem, but no undertaking to question the policies of criminalisation. I have little doubt that if decriminalisation were adopted by the European Union it would prove to be the answer to one of the greatest and most intractable problems of modern society. If somebody with the authority and experience of Father McVerrey, who does so much for the disadvantaged youth of Dublin, makes a plea in the *Irish Times* to decriminalise drugs, we surely should take notice.

DOCTORS AND THE PREVENTION OF DISEASE

In the course of their work, doctors have the opportunity of advising patients about remaining healthy. The knowledge needed to prevent illness and maintain good health has only come in the last generation or two as population research identified the causes of the major chronic illnesses that afflict mankind. We now recognise some of the major influences which contribute to ill-health: alcohol and drug abuse, cigarette smoking, poor eating habits, obesity, lack of exercise and exercise facilities, and mood changes. These causes are few in number and, while they are still all-too-common in Western society, lifestyle changes have contributed to much-improved general heath and longevity. It is right therefore that doctors in the course of practice should be prepared to advise their patients, whether they are sick or not, about the clear road to health and longevity.

However, the major responsibility for providing the framework for good community health rests with the government and the educational authorities. The role of government is to provide suitable facilities for exercise and sport in the community and to encourage a culture where good eating habits are not being prejudiced by the food industry and retailers. Good government must also be aware that investment in education pays rich dividends. In our own research work we have confirmed the findings of others that general education plays a crucial part in influencing people to follow the precepts and example of healthy living. Clearly, our education authorities have an obligation to advance the principles of good physical and mental health. We hear about obesity and the obesity syndrome from all quarters, but many parents remain oblivious of this threat to their children's health and future; and there is little attempt by the government to stem its inexorable progress, despite our politicians' lip service to the matter. Without a proactive government, nothing will be done and we will inevitably catch up to the high prevalence of obesity in America. Education, closely linked to the ability to respond to health advice, is the clearest way forward to improve the health of society, thereby reducing health service costs.

I perceive the principal reason that many clinicians and general practitioners fail to provide adequate lifestyle advice can be attributed to lack of time and their poor training in counselling. Most practising doctors are busy and tend to be under pressure because of time constraints, leaving them little opportunity for the more time-consuming counselling on illness prevention. Thus, it is welcome that the role of prevention in the clinical area is now being taking over by nurses and trained health counselling who have the time and the training as health-promoting members of the healing profession.

Other factors which diminish the role of the practising doctor in the area of prevention are:

- Undergraduate training with little emphasis on the impor tance of epidemiological research aimed at promoting a healthy society.
- Our traditional and vocational commitment to treating the sick.
- Intervention is more personal and immediate or urgent action whereas leisurely counselling is most appreciated by the indi vidual patient.
- The vested interests of hospitals and commercial companies.

However, it is apparent that in countries such as Ireland and the United States, where a two-tier health service prevails, and in other countries providing profit-motivated health care, preventive practices are developing among doctors which raise serious medical and ethical questions and which conflict with the doctor's traditional role of caring for the sick. I have already alluded to the common and undesirable practice of prescribing drugs for healthy people as a measure of avoiding illness. In recent years, there has been an increasing tendency to invite a patient who has recovered from an illness to return to the doctor at regular intervals for 'review' or a 'routine check-up' which maintains the patient on a perpetual medical treadmill.

There is increasing resort by the public to the provision of regular and elaborate physical or executive checks on the healthy. These services are now provided in at least three of our for-profit private hospitals in Ireland and are widely advertised. Some are available in other private clinics. They are aimed at the more wealthy citizens and they are not evidence based by proper trials. This type of service is not provided by our teaching and university hospitals. These executive tests have been criticised in an editorial in the prestigious *New England Journal of Medicine* on three grounds. They are described as expensive, ineffective in improving health and iniquitous; they are not evidence based according to the author.

Tests in healthy people can too often show equivocal or abnormal findings which lead to further tests and further medical intrusion; and a clear bill of health does not preclude the need to adopt a healthy lifestyle if one is to hope for normal health and longevity. The more expensive services of this nature includes a physical examination, which may or may not be thorough, and a number of routine tests which may be impressive to the client but which are not without their own problems. We talk in medical practice about the sensitivity and specificity of a test, that is, if there is anything wrong, will it be always confirmed by the test and, if there is nothing wrong, is the test always normal? The answer in both cases is no. Executive checks should only be approved if they include a discussion with and after a clinical examination by the supervising doctor. In this way the tests provided can be appropriate to the patient and the disadvantages of doing tests can be reduced to a minimum. The difficulties which can arise from doing a battery of tests without clinical indications are less likely to occur.

We are also exposed in Ireland to recent advertisements from a British firm which, for a fee of €169, will carry out four investigations in thirty minutes in a mobile unit without an examination or clinical history. The results will be sent to the client within 21days. This is a most pernicious and intrusive approach and is full of problems, particularly because of the high number of 'abnormalities' which are likely to emerge and which will be treated as pathological or subjected to further investigation by the client's general practitioner. The brochure claims that the client will be informed of the likelihood of a stroke or heart attack on very dubious but, for the lay person, seemingly plausible evidence. This is likely to do considerable harm by causing unnecessary anxiety and by increasing the medicalisation of the public. It is imperative that the health and medical authorities should be aware of the threat this service may hold for the public. I have spoken to the Minister of Health and Children, Mary Harney, and to the head of the HSE about my concern. The Minister has undertaken to deal with my complaint.

The important factor in ensuring the health of our society is public health education. We know the major threats to our health and we are best served by following the advice of NGOs, such as the Irish Heart Foundation or the Irish Cancer Society, and by government through encouragement of healthy lifestyles, and by providing adequate facilities for exercise, sport and social cohesion. It should not be necessary for us to seek tests or unnecessary visits to doctors if we follow the precepts of good physical and mental health. The traditional role of the doctor is to attend to the sick and to follow the precepts of Hippocrates.

12

PUBLIC HEALTH CAMPAIGNS

Soon after the publication of our first paper on the relationship between smoking and heart disease in 1963, I became active in publicising the dangers of cigarette smoking. This was the beginning of an increasingly active public health campaign aimed at the prevention of heart disease and stroke, with particular emphasis on the health consequences of smoking. This involved my increasing prominence in the media and, at the same time, my recurring embarrassment because many of my medical colleagues disapproved of what they called 'publicity'. It was suggested that I was being unethical in promoting myself with the public and that this contravened the ethical guidelines of the Medical Council. I was particularly sensitive when newspapers appeared with banner headlines and some of the rather emotive titles such as 'Top Heart Surgeon Lashes the Ash', as occurred after I had protested publicly about cigarette advertisements at hurling matches.

I have seven well-filled scrapbooks in my library containing cuttings from the national and medical newspapers which leave little doubt that I had become a prominent advocate in the area of health promotion, particularly in relation to smoking, the need for aerobic exercise and the importance of nutrition in relation to heart disease and cancer. A few of my closer colleagues supported me but in general I felt an undercurrent of criticism among my colleagues although seldom expressed in my presence. Many complaints were made by colleagues to the Medical Council, and the Council was obliged to bring these complaints to my notice. There is a rather voluminous correspondence between myself and the Medical Council where I insisted that it was the duty of our profession to protect the public from illness when we had the appropriate information to do so and that the purveyor of the information should be identified to confirm the authenticity of the advice. At no time did I receive the approval of the Medical Council – but my replies made the point that, if any action were taken against me by the Council, the High Court would confirm that my actions were not only legal but essential in relation to public health. Hence, all formal reproaches from the Medical Council were silenced, but this did not prevent some colleagues raising the issue in a discussion at a meeting of the Irish Medical Association in 1970, under the title 'Doctors and the Media'.

The panel on the platform included the president of the Medical Council, Professor Mitchell, Professor Tom Murphy, President of University College, Dublin and former Dean of its medical faculty; John Healy, correspondent for the *Irish Times*; the editor of the *British Medical Journal* and Dr Harry Counihan, respiratory physician and editor of the *Irish Medical Journal*. They showed little sympathy for the critics and agreed that those with the necessary qualifications could – and should – speak in public about health matters. It was generally agreed that doctors should avoid referring to medical issues which brought attention to the doctor's own private practice.

Despite my sensitivity, I was unable to resist the compulsion to speak out on public health issues when the circumstances called for comment, perhaps because of my political background. As to the charge of seeking publicity to attract patients, being involved in writing, in public speaking, in giving lectures and in being involved with Heart Foundation and Irish Medical Association activities left limited time for private practice. At the same time, critics and 'competitors' were sitting at home beside the telephone and freely available to those who wished to avail of their services.

My public activities included appearances on television. They included four appearances on *The Late Late Show* with the inimitable Gay Byrne. One was on cigarette smoking; the second was on exercise, and on this occasion we both demonstrated our cycling abilities on bicycle ergometers in the studio. If I recall correctly, Gay fell off his bike! A third was on the health consequences of high-fat foods and cholesterol, and the fourth on health aspects of salt. I am still reminded many years later by viewers of the salt interview that the programme had some influence in leading to the later reduction in salt consumption by the public and its use by the food industry. I was afterwards contacted by a senior representative of the salt industry who seemed greatly concerned by my reference to excess salt as a cause of high blood pressure and stomach cancer. His response was sympathetic and understanding. The many comments I received after the television programmes were a reminder of how effective television is as a means of communication.

The sensible reaction of the salt industry was unlike the adversarial reaction of the dairy industry, and some of their prominent medical advisors, to my third appearance on *The Late Late Show* on the subject of cholesterol and the nutritional basis of coronary heart disease. What should we advise about maintaining a normal cholesterol profile? We should eat a balanced diet; no food is harmful if eaten in reasonable quantities, but we need to encourage more fruit and vegetables, fish and carbohydrate foods rather than meat and dairy foods. If the world were committed to a fruit and vegetable instead of a meat-focused food economy, it would benefit the health of society as well as providing more food to support a huge and expanding human population. It would also reduce the harmful methane emissions, a highly significant contributor to climate change.

The leaders of the dairy industry in Ireland and the UK were hostile to our campaign and were misled by their medical advisors on the cholesterol issue. The industry was initially in denial and fought back vigorously. The director of the Dairy Board was their principal spokesman in this country and he, my colleagues and I had an exchange of letters, which was published in the press. We were able to report the evidence implicating saturated fat and cholesterol in contributing to the coronary epidemic. This evidence was supported by hundreds of research reports, by at least twenty commissions appointed by governments and international medical organisations, and by all the heart foundations which then existed. The director of the Dairy Board was only able to quote the views of one 'distinguished' nutritionist in the United States.

A controversial RTÉ documentary programme on heart disease in the late 1970s, *In Vegas It's Called Odds*, was being marketed in the United States. Its purpose was to throw doubt on the role of cholesterol in the genesis of coronary disease. It rightly provoked a strong protest in the Irish news media over alleged financing by the National Dairy Council and being marketed despite the views of WHO and the heart foundation. I wrote to the press accusing the programme makers of bias and distortion of the facts about heart disease. Surely, in situations like this, where an industry perceives itself as being under threat by public policies, its representatives should interview all agencies, including responsible government departments, before introducing ill-informed and contentious arguments which ultimately prove to be futile and counterproductive to their own perceived interests.

It was a year or two later that I, representing the Irish Heart Foundation, met with the CEOs of the major dairy companies to remind them that the Irish industry would lose out to foreign competitors if it ignored the health significance of foods low in saturated fat. This followed a letter I had published in the *Irish Times* which had received editorial support. They were soon to respond, particularly to increasing public anxiety about heart disease and to the looming threat from the Flora group and other well-publicised international food industries which were providing increasingly popular and acceptable low-saturated-fat spreads and foods.

Of course it still left a number of conservative colleagues who, for one reason or another, continued to be critical of our views on the nutritional aspects of heart disease and who remained in denial. They included prominent leaders of the profession who were experts in their own fields and sometimes well known to the public, but who had little insight into the power and potential of epidemiological research in establishing causes of the chronic diseases of mankind.

Sir John McMichael, for example, was the senior physician in the renowned Hammersmith Hospital in London. He was one of the influential physicians in the UK who was provocatively outspoken in his criticism of the view that nutrition and an abnormal cholesterol profile were important in the genesis of the arterial disease which led to coronary heart disease and stroke. His article in the *British Medical Journal* was published in March 1979, and it evoked a detailed response in the correspondence columns from Noel Hickey, Ian Graham and myself. However, with his prestige and our relatively obscure provincial origins, it is unnecessary to add that his intervention would further delay the adoption of measures to reduce the high rate of mortality from heart disease in the UK and elsewhere. Like other prominent critics of our health promotion strategies in both the UK and Ireland, he had no training in medical epidemiology and no conception of the huge value to be gained from studies of populations when seeking to identify the causes of chronic disease.

Another colleague of his in the Hammersmith Hospital, who was a prominent member of the British Cardiac Society, frequently referred disparagingly to me and two of my colleagues in the society when we presented papers on aspects of prevention. He once said to me, 'You cannot prevent heart disease. You can only treat it!' The Hammersmith doctors were perceived as the leaders of cardiology in Britain – and they certainly were leaders in the diagnosis and surgical treatment of congenital and heart valve disease and in developing the heart/lung machine – and, although trained scientists, they were capable of making categorical statements about the results of epidemiological research about which they had little knowledge. The strong anti-prevention role of British cardiologists had an important and adverse effect in delaying health promotion in that country, which obviously affected Irish opinion as well.

Similarly, some of the academics in the department of preventive medicine in certain of our universities were in denial about the importance of cholesterol in the genesis of heart disease and, surprisingly, one prominent member rejected cigarette smoking as a health hazard. The academics were supported by other prominent members of my profession in Ireland, including at least one professor of medicine. When these critics, however eminent in their own speciality, become involved in areas outside their own expertise, they tend to be dogmatic in their assertions and to use more emotive language than the more muted and restrained words of the epidemiologist, whose training is based on the principles of evidence and on seeking the truth. They tend to be dismissive of their colleagues, a reaction which would never occur among colleagues of the same discipline who might differ on some aspect particular to their speciality. I have in my files an extraordinary collection of statements from such colleagues – that coronary disease was simply the result of ageing or that 60 percent of cases of heart attack were genetic in origin, a statement totally inconsistent with our own and international epidemiological research.

Because of our public pronouncements about the need to eat healthy food, one cardiologist in Dublin warned the public about the dangers of developing mass neurosis about health in relation to nutrition; this in the early 1980s when I estimated that of the £3 billion health budget, only 0.2 percent was earmarked by the government for preventive strategies. The question of inducing individual or national neurosis as a result of health education was a recurring theme during these years. In response to an article in the medical press by one of our better-known psychiatrists in Dublin, who thought that the epidemiologists denied the virtues of treatment, I said that we accept the importance and the interdependence of both disciplines. He was critical of what he saw as our exclusive commitment to prevention, but it was the exclusive commitment to treatment of most doctors was the real problem. I am not aware of anyone who fully denies the value of treatment.

SMOKING

Smoking loomed large in my pronouncements during those years. Among my colleagues there was for too long a general indifference to discouraging patients from the habit. Patients admitted with exacerbations of bronchitis and pneumonia were being discharged without being advised to stop smoking, only to soon return to the wards. Smoking was allowed in the wards and there was no expertise in counselling patients and the public about discontinuing the habit or to warn about the likelihood of recidivism after stopping. And such counselling does require patience and expertise as we were to learn during our very active smoking control programmes.

The media too were largely indifferent to the anti-smoking campaign and one prominent newspaper refused to accept anti-smoking articles or letters for a long period. The cigarette industry wisely kept close to the ground; it avoided controversy, at least in Ireland, and only budged when legislation forced changes in the composition of the cigarette and in the circumstances of their sale. There were other forces gathering to highlight the adverse effect of cigarette smoking on health – mounting taxation (resisted by the trade unions) and voluntary health groups, such as Irish Ash, supported by the Cancer Society and the Heart Foundation, and the education section of the Department of Health – but generally not by our political masters.

Gradually from the late 1960s the number of smokers began to fall; the proportion of smokers among men had dropped from more 70 percent to about 24 percent in 2004. This decline over the years has had a dramatic effect on the incidence of the smoking-related diseases, with a substantial and continuing increase in longevity. The reduction is also notable in coronary disease, stroke and respiratory disease, and international research confirms that almost 50 percent of the recent improvement in longevity in Western countries can be attributed to the decline of cigarette smoking among the middle-aged. The decline of smoking is having a greater influence on longevity than one might expect because it is mostly the young who continue to smoke and they are still within a low-risk group because of their shorter exposure to tobacco. In fact, in 2009 it was reported that the number of smokers has risen to 27 percent in both sexes. It is likely that this increase has been largely among young people.

Mícheál Martin's decision to ban smoking in public was an inspired response to pressure from our NGOs and individual activists, who have continued to plead the cause of the public's wellbeing. Our politicians have in general been slow in the past to face the tobacco industry, the retailers, the smokers and the trade unions, but special mention must be made of Charles Haughey's early and unsuccessful attempts to convince a reluctant cabinet to ban cigarette advertising. At the time I had this to say in a letter to the *Irish Times*:

> I am reminded of the occasion in the summer of 1984 when snide remarks about the Minister for Health and his efforts to encourage community control of smoking were made by the chairman of one of our tobacco companies. At the time he was presenting the trophy to the winner of the tobacco-sponsored international golf competition held at Royal Dublin. His remarks were greeted with applause. Surely this spontaneous reaction on the part of the onlookers does not represent the considered view on the Irish public.

For those of us who lived forty or more years ago and who remember the everpresence of the cigarette and its inherent part in the day-to-day life in Ireland, it is difficult to comprehend the magnitude of the change in our environment and in our social and domestic habits that was brought about over the years culminating in Míchéal Martin's historic legislation.

While our research at St Vincent's Hospital included all aspects of heart disease causation, treatment and prevention, we had a particular interest and research involvement in smoking, in its role as a major cause of multi-system disease, in counselling our patients and the public in discouraging the habit, and in understanding its social, political and economic implications. During the 1970s up to the early 1990s after my retirement, we published numerous research reports about smoking in the national and international medical press based on the St Vincent's Heart Study, which continued from 1965 until 2006. Among our publications, our report in the *British Heart Journal* in 1983 confirmed the results of smoking cessation on patients' long-term survival and on further symptoms and complications. We were the first in the world (at the same time as colleagues in Sweden) to report the dramatic reduction in mortality of patients who had survived a heart attack and who had stopped smoking compared with those who continued to smoke. We were also the first to publish the results of the coronary risk factors in women in the leading American heart journal, *Circulation*, in 1967and to find that they shared the same risk factors as men; that is, cigarette smoking, high blood cholesterol and high blood pressure.

We also questioned the hypothesis that women inherently live longer than men because of their genetic makeup. A research study published by us in the *American Journal of Public Health* in 1970 of the male and female smoking habits in fifteen different countries where the necessary data were available about cigarette consumption and about mortality showed that cigarette consumption was the major factor in accounting for the life expectancy discrepancy between the sexes. During the period of the study, smoking among women was much less common than among men. We concluded:

> Our results are consistent with the hypothesis that cigarette smoking, because of its association with coronary heart disease

and other chronic disorders, may partly or completely account for the better female compared to male life expectancy experienced over the last fifty years.

Gender mortality is now beginning to converge as smoking among women has increased in recent years and has shown a marked decrease in middle-aged men. The discrepancy was only 0.3 years in Ireland 104 years ago when there was little cigarette smoking among the population; and despite the certainty that men were at greater risk than women because of occupation, army service, alcohol consumption and a greater tendency to risk-taking. The disparity between the sexes at birth peaked in Ireland at 5.7 years in 1986 but had converged by 0.8 years by 2005, according to the latest Central Statistics Office report. The discrepancy will narrow further as male and female lifestyles become more similar.

We reported in the *American Journal of Clinical Nutrition* in 1973 that, with proper counselling, patients could be induced to stop smoking without an increase in weight, a common fear of smokers considering quitting. We recorded public and professional attitudes to cigarette smoking, and the effect of cigar and pipe smoking on heart disease. Many other papers dealt with smoking as part of the broader aspects of heart disease, its natural history and its causes.

We set up a special counselling service to encourage patients to stop smoking. Nicotine is recognised as the most addictive drug known, hence the difficulties involved in stopping smoking and the frequency of recidivism. Addiction exists when we have difficulty in making firm decisions about stopping and where immediate deprivation leads to physiological and psychological side-effects of withdrawal which may prove intolerable. I learnt a lot from my own experience which provided the insights to understand the problems of other smokers. I stopped cigarette smoking at the age of 37 but only after ten or more years of attempting to stop. I was helped eventually to overcome the habit by becoming a dedicated and committed squash player with a different addiction, strenuous exercise.

In our follow-up of patients we were able to report in the *British Medical Journal* in 1983 a long-term quit rate of more than 60 percent in our subjects, a level far above the results reported from other centres. This success rate was only achieved by an understanding of the difficulties in stopping and the factors which are most likely to achieve lasting cessation and to prevent recidivism. Many were also helped by having had a cigarette related illness. We were assisted by using specially-designed literature to inform and to encourage our patients, and we were not slow to warn the recalcitrant of the likely consequences of further smoking.

The campaign against smoking in the western world was largely conducted by NGOs such as heart and cancer foundations, and by dedicated individuals and a few dedicated medical groups. Many more years would pass after the early 1960s before doctors, cardiologists and lung specialists were to take active steps to discourage smoking among their patients. The delay in action against the cigarette is a measure of the vested interests of the tobacco industry, the power of money and advertising in a free market, the smokers themselves, the trade unions, the retailers and the publicans, not to mention poorly motivated politicians and a conservative medical profession. It was to take forty years after the US Surgeon General's seminal report in 1964 before Ireland took the decision to ban smoking in public places. It was a time of widespread denial among doctors and the public.

Of course there were isolated reports about the association between cigarette smoking and respiratory disease before the College of Physicians report appeared in 1963 and the Surgeon General's in 1964, but these were ignored. Indeed, the first protests against tobacco can be attributed to King James I in England, whose famed assault against tobacco was encapsulated in a thirteen line 'sonnet' attributed (retrospectively) to William Shakespeare:

> Fair fragrant weed, late from Virginia brought,
> Thy smoke evokes a heavenly content,
> And brings to woeful wight with toil forspent
> Tranquillity and sessions of sweet thought.
> Yet speaks our liege, our learned Scots dynast,
> Affirming poisons do those leaves contain
> That rot men's lungs and breed anginal pain.
> Tobacco damns he with his counterblast!
> Shall smokers name in centuries to come

King James the wisest fool in Christendom?
Or doth he seek with seers divining eyes
A siren Nicotina, seeking tears,
A usurer who charges men in years?

At least Mr Martin, our late minister for health, can be complimented for his initiative and his positive response to our three anti-tobacco NGOs, but I believe that there was little choice in the long run because the evidence was emerging about the adverse effect of passive smoking on health and the looming threat of litigation by non-smokers with cancer and heart disease who claimed to have been exposed to passive smoking. The politicians may be slow to confront vested interests on some issues which are deemed desirable for our society but in the case of the cigarette, when the question of litigation loomed, the writing was on the wall. The earliest legislation to ban smoking in public was in the US in 1975 when the Minnesota Clean Indoor Air Act was passed by the Minnesota State Legislature.

Peter Taylor, in his book, *Smoke Ring: The Politics of Tobacco*, wrote that it would require an act of rare political courage on the part of a politician to confront the tobacco industry. Charles Haughey, who as minister for health in the Jack Lynch administration in the 1970s gave our research work major financial support, was an exception. He was anxious to ban all tobacco advertising but received no support from his colleagues in cabinet. The great majority of politicians showed little inclination to oppose the tobacco barons. They did at times introduce appropriate legislation to control the worst excesses of the tobacco industry, but they and their civil servants and local authority officials did little or nothing to enforce such legislation.

Mícheál Martin's 2004 initiative was very successful and has been largely and even enthusiastically accepted by the Irish population. It confirms how legislation can be effective if firmly enforced by authority. It has abruptly changed a society which was dominated by the smoking habit to one where we seldom think or even remember the days of the ubiquitous cigarette and its influence in our social lives and, indeed, its bonding effect on friendships.

In my earlier days, the small Woodbines were mostly smoked by the working classes, as they were then described, while Player's Navy Cut and Will's Gold Flake were preferred by the better-off. Later there was a penchant among men for stronger cigarettes, such as Churchman and Capstan Full Strength, and even for the more exotic such as the French Galois and the Turkish-scented Balkan Sobranie. Cigarettes were generally smoked down to the shortest butt, but not infrequently, especially among students, a part was saved to enjoy later.

When I was a student and resident at St Vincent's Hospital, one of my bedroom colleagues kept an old battered Capstan cigarette tin beside his bed. In it he kept a collection of cigarette butts, collected from various ashtrays and from the floor during the day. Two or three times during the night he would wake, extract a butt from the tin, light up and take a few drags, and then turn over to sleep again. He was one of the most uncommunicative people I have ever met and one of the most addicted to nicotine. He subsequently went to Northern Ireland where he was a general practitioner in County Armagh. Not surprisingly, he was reported to have died from lung cancer in his early forties.

While patently obvious to us now, there appeared to be little awareness of the devastating effect of cigarette smoking on health and premature mortality at that time, apart from the Dublin jackeen's description of the poor man's Woodbines as 'coffin nails'! It was well into the early 1960s, with the publication of the Royal College of Physicians and Surgeon General's reports, before there was any suspicion that smoking was a serious health threat and the widespread acceptance of the adverse effects of cigarettes was to wait many more years, even within the medical profession. There was a sense of denial about the harmful effects of the cigarette and there were several reasons why this was so. With up to 70 percent of men smoking, there were insufficient non-smokers to make a meaningful comparison which, added to by the supposed benign nature of pipe smoking, may have delayed the proper appreciation of the harmful effects of cigarettes. Mass denial appears to be part of the human condition, as existed in Ireland during the Celtic Tiger and as currently exists about environmental destruction and the population explosion.

Life expectancy among the professional and business middle classes in Ireland, represented by the membership of my golf club, has increased dramatically over the past fifty years, largely because cigarette smoking is now very unusual amongst the members. The consumption of alcohol has also moderated, at least among the male members (but perhaps not among women), but the fog of smoke, the well-filled ashtray, the acrid smell and the scattered evidence of the smoking habit are no longer with us. It is a measure of the improved life expectation that, in 1957, I was one of sixteen past captains alive; by the year 2008 there were thirty-four alive. In 1957, life expectancy was such that we had few honorary members, that is, those who had been members for forty years or more; by 1998 this category was abolished because of the excessive number of non-paying honorary members.

Some of the physicians and all the surgeons at St Vincent's Hospital were smokers in the mid- and late-1940s. They smoked during ward rounds and it was the ward sister's privilege to carry the ashtray. Remarkably, two of the surgeons for whom I administered anaesthetics in 1946 smoked regularly *during* operations. They were enabled to do so by the assistance of the theatre sister, who would light the cigarette and hold it in a Spencer Wells forceps. With a nod, the surgeon would turn his head, the sister would pull down the mask, hold the cigarette to his lips in the forceps; he would take a drag or two, and inhale the smoke deeply into his lungs. I assume the falling ash was no problem, being certainly aseptic and therefore unlikely to damage the exposed tissues! Many of the consultant doctors I knew at the Mater and St Vincent's Hospital in the 1940s and 1950s died prematurely from lung cancer, stroke, heart disease or emphysema, as did many of the middle-aged male members of my golf club.

The 1950s and 1960s was the time of silver cigarette cases and ornate cigarette and cigar boxes. The cigarette holder was also common, particularly among women smokers. The long artistic model conveyed an elegance and sophistication. The holder was useful in reducing the nicotine staining on the hands and the upper lip. The American cigarettes had not yet invaded Europe or these islands, although Camels were known to us and were the first cigarettes to arrive with the American troops in the North during the war. Later Camels were advertised as either 'smoked by doctors' or 'approved by doctors', thus no doubt implying their health virtues. The liberal supply of cigarettes to the American troops gave a fillip to the cigarette smoking habits worldwide and I expect that more American soldiers were eventually to die prematurely from smoking rather than from the results of battle.

The 1950s and 1960s was a time when the sharing of cigarettes was the social norm, the offering of a cigarette was an essential part of social intercourse (and, not infrequently, after sexual intercourse!). It was still a sophisticated habit despite the heavy fog at social gatherings and the chronic, productive smoker's cough – 'the sound of mucous', as one cynic said – later to be identified as the harbinger of lung cancer. The pervasive cigarette ash and collection of butts were part of our normal environment, as were cigarette burns on tables, chairs, upholstery and clothing. I lost several trousers and suits by dropping ash while smoking in the car. It was the time of the charred and nicotine-stained fingers; the flat, penetrating and pungent smell of nicotine off one's clothes and in the house. There were no filter tips then and so the tar content was much greater. It was the time of the chain-smoker who smoked right through the day and night, lighting one cigarette after another, and of the diner who smoked between courses. In Ireland as in Britain, it was the time of the short butt, so that none of the precious tobacco could be wasted. Like the last few drops of Guinness, the last drag was the best, even if it was to prove the most carcinogenic.

It was the time when so many middle-aged people died unexpectedly and without warning from the 'acute indigestion' described by the media, later to be identified as the common form of heart attack, a myocardial infarction or coronary thrombosis. Sudden unexpected death was common a generation or more ago – on the golf course, in the football stadium, the street, in bed and elsewhere – when cigarette smoking was a widespread habit. The forensic evidence available to us now confirms that sudden, unexpected death is now less common in Ireland and I have had very few reports of such an event in my two golf clubs in recent years. I have already referred to the chain smoking bridge players in the Regent Bridge Club.

The sophistication of the smoking habit was particularly evident in films in these early years. At every hiatus in a film, the hero would produce a slim silver cigarette case, and, carefully choosing a cigarette, would tap it lightly, light it with some little ceremony, and perhaps offer one to the heroine, all designed to attract our attention and our admiration. The film makers were paid by the tobacco companies to provide these intimate scenes. I recall two leading stars travelling by train through the Rockies in a particularly romantic film. The hero carefully chose two cigarettes, lit both and handed one to the heroine whose happy smile and flashing eyes conveyed the ultimate in pleasure and anticipation.

The smoker's cough, shortness of breath and the production of phlegm identified smokers who were particularly prone to developing emphysema or lung cancer. The smoking diseases were dose related as measured by the number of years smoking, the number of cigarettes consumed, the degree of inhalation and the size of the remaining butt. It was the norm for some heavy smokers to suffer from severe and prolonged coughing in the morning with the production of copious quantities of phlegm and possibly too with nausea or a tendency to vomiting.

The industry's denial and corruption has been well described in many well-researched books, such as Peter Taylor's *Smoke Ring* and Ian Gately's *La Diva Nicotina*. The industry did everything possible to discredit the US Surgeon General and many medical institutions. Their attacks referred to the unreliability of statistics, despite their crucial role in medical research. The American government was also responsible for the industry's incursion into many third world countries where the nationally-controlled tobacco industries were frequently destroyed by American advertising. American aid was offered at the price of admitting the well-known American brands. One sees the Marlboro placards and bills everywhere, including the poorest countries.

The legal profession has had a field day in terms of the fees they have earned. Both those who appeared on behalf of the industry and those who acted for patients and governments earned between them many billions of dollars. According to Ian Gately, lawyers in Florida earned an average of $233 million each. Nor were doctors entirely blameless: Lucky Strikes were advertised as being good because they reduced appetite and prevented obesity. They solicited the opinions of American doctors, offering them five cartons of Lucky Strike cigarettes. According to Gately, 20,679 doctors endorsed the brand as 'healthy'. Surely the ethics and greed of the commercial, professional and personal worlds must reflect an inherent part of human nature.

13

THE IRISH HEART FOUNDATION

My interest in the causes and the prevention of coronary disease was to lead to my proposal in 1965 to the Irish Cardiac Society that we set up an Irish heart foundation aimed at bringing lay people as well as medical professionals together in dealing with the coronary epidemic and with associated conditions such as stroke. I was on the committee of the British Cardiac Society at the time and was fully informed about the setting-up of the British Heart Foundation, which was established in the early 1960s. My proposal was fully supported by the Irish Cardiac Society and led to establishing a working group with members from the Society and a number of lay people whom I had suggested as being suitable. Some of those were members of my golf club who were influential in the business life of the country and others were prominent in the public service and in industry. Things moved fairly quickly and by June of 1966 we had the official launch of the Irish Heart Foundation at Jury's Hotel in Dublin, attended by the President, Éamon de Valera, the Taoiseach Seán Lemass, the Minister for Health Donnacha O'Malley and by distinguished colleagues from abroad including Paul White, representing the American Heart Association, and Graham Hayward, representing the British Cardiac Society.

Overcoming the financial problems posed the greatest challenge for the working group but, after much discussion, the decision was made to employ professional fundraisers. The concept of professional fundraising had only recently arrived in Ireland and was first employed by Clongowes Wood College. The Irish Heart Foundation was the second organisation to avail of this form of funding. Within a year of launching, we raised enough funds to buy No. 4 Clyde Road as headquarters for £16,000 and to appoint a full-time director with a modest support staff. The foundation was housed for its first year in the garden flat of 3 Clyde Road which was in the joint ownership of my colleague Oliver McCullen and me. I need hardly say that many thought us extravagant to pay such a big price for No. 4 in 1967, particularly as the adjoining No. 3 had been acquired by Oliver and me two years earlier for £12,000! When we reached the halcyon days of the Celtic Tiger in 2006, its worth had increased about four hundred-fold, to about €8 million!

Shortly after the Foundation was established, the highly successful mobile Mediscan programme was conceived and began operation. It was organised under the direction of my colleague Noel Hickey, who became the medical director of the foundation. Noel was active in promoting the health policies of the foundation, in training our many loyal and devoted nurses and in doing so much valuable epidemiological work. Ian Graham, who was later to become President of the foundation, and David Kilcoyne also contributed their share of energy and expertise to the success of the foundation in its early days.

Mediscan was organised in a specially-designed mobile caravan and covered almost the entire country during subsequent years and remained active with a high profile until 1994. The screening programme was conducted by nurses and included a blood pressure check, cholesterol estimation, a smoking and aerobic exercise history, and a weight check. Apart from the beneficial effect Mediscan had on individual behaviour, it was a valuable reminder to the profession about the feasibility of the preventive approach to heart disease. It was the first glimmerings of campaigns to encourage healthy living and it coincided with the beginning of a real improvement in the life expectancy of the Irish population.

My colleagues Sean Blake, Gerry Gearty, Conor Ward and Barry O'Donnell joined me on the working group which set up the foundation. Gerry Gearty, in association with the inimitable Noel Gleeson, played the principal role in organising a most successful mobile coronary care service which served the city of Dublin well for years. This service was established shortly after a similar system was organised in Belfast by Frank Pantridge. Our system had the advantage over Belfast in dispensing with the doctor in the ambulance and relying on permanent, highly-trained ambulance personnel. The service, which played a major role in saving lives and in publicising the urgency of dealing with the coronary epidemic, was terminated because of lack of funds, caused by the failure of the local health authorities to pay for the less affluent citizens.

The foundation organised hypertension detection clinics countrywide at supermarket outlets and community centres, again designed by Noel Hickey. Like Mediscan, this was staffed by trained nurses. Information about desirable lifestyle changes was included as part of the process. These clinics commenced in the early 1970s. The foundation's activities confirmed the important role nurses and other paramedical professions have in health promotional activities. By 2008, much of the preventive and rehabilitation services in cardiology are carried out by nurses, nutritionists and social workers. It is largely because of them that a much more comprehensive service is now available to our patients.

Much has happened since these early days. We now have a vibrant organisation with links to the Irish Cancer Society, the Health Services Executive, and the Health Promotion Unit of the Department of Health and Children, ASH and with other NGOs. This expanding network is playing an important part in improving the health of the Irish people, as exemplified by our national smoking control policies and the adoption of healthier lifestyles, particularly among the educated. Yet more needs to be done by our NGOs and government in relation to aerobic exercise facilities and to reverse the steady rise of obesity. On these two issues the government has been vocal at times, but less than active in following the foundation's concerns about the looming obesity problem. Above all, much needs to be done in the realm of general health education and public facilities for exercise. The Heart Foundation, with its many committees dealing with various aspects of heart disease prevention and treatment, and its full support of the medical profession and the public, can be proud of the part it has played in leading the current reduction in heart disease and stroke mortality, and in the dramatic increase in life expectancy which we have witnessed in the last forty years.

Éamon de Valera agreed to accept patronage of the foundation after I called to the Áras to explain the purpose of the new organisation. He was graciousness itself in giving me twenty minutes of his time. He greeted me at the door of his study with the *cúpla focail* – *Conas tá d'athair?* ('How is your father?') – and he parted with me at the end of the twenty-minute interval with *Is dócha go bhuil tú pósta?* ('I suppose you are married?')(I was then forty-four years old) and when I replied in the affirmative he said, *Is dócha go bhuil páistí agat?* ('I suppose you have children?') He had just handed me a cheque for £100 for the foundation – a generous gift from him, as was his agreeing to act as patron of the foundation for he explained that, as president of Ireland, he intended to confine his patronage to the Irish Red Cross and then only because he had been its patron for many years before his elevation to head of state.

The decision of the Irish Heart Foundation to confine its early policies to health promotion and disease prevention was unique among foundations worldwide. Other foundations put the emphasis on support for clinical research and service rather than on public health promotion. The American Heart Association was unusual in that, from an early stage, it supported in equal measure clinical research and service. It was the example of the American policy that encouraged us to adopt the preventive approach, particularly because of our limited resources and the looming coronary epidemic. Although we were successful in our fundraising from the beginning, our resources were limited and in the earlier years could not stretch to assisting clinical research and services. Our policy was particularly appropriate in a small country such as Ireland. Costly cardiovascular research could be left to bigger and more affluent centres abroad; while Ireland, with its stable population and good communication infrastructure, was a suitable area for public health education, prevention and population research.

The epidemiological research undertaken by the foundation was related to finding causes, to the proper approach to effective education and to studying factors which determine successful compliance to desirable lifestyle changes in the population.

Our early policies in this regard were not popular with some of our colleagues who thought that the foundation should be encouraging clinical services and research rather than espousing public health information. But in hindsight, and because of Ireland's suitability for epidemiological research, we certainly made the correct decision at the time. Other colleagues objected to the Mediscan programme and the hypertension clinics, believing that it was supplanting the role of the family doctor. However, critics were few and would eventually subscribe to the work of the foundation.

THE KILKENNY HEALTH PROJECT

Finland had the highest incidence of coronary disease in the world in the 1960s and 1970s, most evident in the North Karelia province. In 1972 the North Karelia Project was established to identify the causes of the epidemic and to reduce the high incidence of the disease. The project had full support from the profession, the public and the government in Helsinki. An intensive public campaign of health promotion was launched and the efficacy of the campaign was compared to the trends in coronary disease in the neighbouring province of Kuopio. The North Karelia Project was an outstanding example of the success of such an extensive and well supported health promoting programme. Finland now has a coronary mortality which is below the average of the Northern European countries.

The Irish Heart foundation decided to emulate the Finnish project by setting up the Kilkenny Health Project in 1985. A committee was formed, of which I was chairman, and advice was sought from two Finnish epidemiologists who travelled to Ireland to assist in defining the objectives and structure of the programme. We were fortunate to have Dr Emer Shelley as director of the project. She had qualified in Trinity College and had had a long training in epidemiology and preventive medicine. To compare the results of the health campaign which was planned for Kilkenny, we compared our results to similar findings in the reference county of Offaly. It is not possible to estimate the influence of the Kilkenny project on the decline in coronary and stroke mortality, but by 1992, when the project ended, there had been a clear and continuous decline in mortality from these conditions in the Republic. Eight papers were subsequently published by Emer Shelley and her co-workers in the national and international press which reported on various aspects of the project and a final report was lodged with the Department of Health.

During the programme, subjects were encouraged to grow their own vegetables and fruit. This met with little success and one resident who was encouraged to do so demurred, thinking such an activity might be perceived as a sign of poverty! It is an odd reflection that counties such as Kilkenny and Wexford, which invariably had fruit and vegetables in their gardens and farms fifty and more years ago, are now entirely dependent on the local supermarket for these items. Every farm in Wexford, a county I have known well since the 1930s, had an orchard. You can still see the lichen-covered stumps of the apple and pear trees close to the farmhouses there. Vegetables were few in variety – cabbage, carrots and onions as well as the potato – but they were widely grown and plentiful.

The Medico-social Research Board

The Medico-social Research Board was established in 1966 at the behest of the then-Minister of Health, Erskine Childers. Dr Geoffrey Dean, a physician and well-known and outstanding medical epidemiologist, was appointed its director and remained in this position until his retirement in 1984. He was assisted by a board of management which included a number of prominent citizens in the medical, social and administrative fields. I was a member during the entire time of its existence. The concept was an inspirational one and much was achieved by the director and the board despite a very modest budget and the huge social and drug problems which existed in the city at that time. Despite its great success on a very limited budget, the life of the board came to an unexpected and unfortunate end in 1986, again at the behest of the then-minister, Barry Desmond. We were subsumed into the newly reorganised Health Research Board whose policies were earlier largely related to clinical and basic research. Those of us who were familiar with the neglect of health promotion by our clinical colleagues were only too well-aware of the poor support epidemiology was likely to receive from its new masters. None of the board members of the MSRB were invited to join the board of the Health Research Board. Despite many protests to Mr Desmond and despite the MSRB's record, we got little satisfaction from the authorities. Some of the achievements of the board and its director are recorded in Dr Dean's autobiography, *The Turnstone: A Doctor's Story* published in 1988. The termination of the life of the MSRB seemed at the time as a confirmation of the government's poor commitment to social research and health promotion.

THE HEALTH PROMOTING HOSPITAL

The Health Promoting Hospitals movement, of which I was the first chairman, was formally established in Ireland in the early 1990s. This organisation has made slow progress here despite Anne O'Riordan, who has led the organisation from the start but whose energies and initiatives have been constrained by inadequate support from a stingy government. Its influence has been important but not as widely effective as it could be. It needs more encouragement from hospital authorities, the HSE and government. Doctors, nurses and other health personnel should be encouraged to include health counselling through practice and training. One euro invested in the HPH movement would be worth ten or more euros invested in our conventional hospital services. St Vincent's Hospital has been an exception, where a counselling service as has been available since 1974 with the creation of the Department of Health Promotion and Prevention in that year.

14

THE IRISH MEDICAL ASSOCIATION AND THE HEALTH SERVICE

I expect that my membership of the IMA and my long-standing interest in the health service was an expression of my political background. I worked closely with two colleagues; Harry Counihan, a respiratory physician from the Richmond Hospital, and William O'Dwyer, a nephrologist in Jervis Street Hospital. As three consultants elected for some years to the Association, we had considerable influence and, being also members of the same golf club, it was said that IMA policy was decided every Sunday morning in Milltown Golf Club! The IMA was not a trade union and we were strenuously opposed to such a role. Apart from any professional function the IMA had in safeguarding the privileges of our profession, its members had a considerable interest in the health and hospital services, and in the country's social services.

Our journal was edited by Counihan and I chaired the publication committee. I also chaired a working party appointed in 1974 which recommended a one-tier compulsory insurance hospital service, which was recommended to the government but ignored by the political and health service authorities. Its acceptance would have been the best answer to our hospital problems and would have avoided many of the organisational and ethical difficulties which persist to this day. The one-tier system remains the best for this country in terms of equality, ethics and efficiency; but the two-tiered profit-motivated and iniquitous system introduced by Mary Harney and the Fianna Fáil administration won the day for our 'Boston' inspired politicians and the indifference of my own profession. She was clearly more influenced by the American rather than the European approach to health delivery services. Her radical changes to the health service were made without any consultation with the medical professions, economists, appropriate public institutions or the members of the Dáil. No white paper, no advisory commission; a step inspired by the same form of capitalist economics which was, just a few years later, to destroy the economic fabric of the country.

In the May and June 1959 issues of the Fine Gael monthly journal of current affairs, the *National Observer*, I wrote two articles about the problems and possible solutions of the health services in Ireland. I advised that health administration should be representative of all appropriate interests and should be removed from the milieu of party politics: I envisaged an authority constituted along the same lines of our semi-State or semi-autonomous bodies. It should also bear the responsibility for the direction of new health policy and should be answerable to the Government on matters of finance.

I believed the health service was weighed down with anomalies and inefficiencies, it lacked a coordinated focus, its shortcomings were aggravated by political influences at national and local levels, the Department of Health and local health authorities shared much of the blame, and the views of the medical profession were ignored in relation to policy and performance. *Plus ça change?* My one hopeful comment referred to the success of the Voluntary Health Insurance which had been established in 1966, three years earlier.

During visits to the United States, I studied aspects of their health delivery system. I was particularly interested in the Kaiser Permanente system which was set up originally in Oakland, California and which has spread to a number of contiguous states. Details of the system are included in my book, *Is the Health Service for Healing?*, published in 2006.

This ninety-six-page monograph on our health service was my response to Ms Harney's proposal to retain a two-tier system of health care and to build a number of for-profit private hospitals on the sites of our public hospitals. It was a plea to organise an equitable one-tier system based on our public hospital services and for compulsory health insurance for all our citizens. I dealt in detail with the current problems prevailing within the current hospital system which included our iniquitous two-tier system, the for-profit private hospitals, the excessive influence of local interests and the numbers of small hospitals. I advocated better organisation of the hospital doctors, including audit and accountability, and encouraging doctors and nurses to participate in administration.

Is the Health Service for Healing? was sent to the 226 deputies and the 60 senators in Dáil Éireann. I received five acknowledgements. It was also sent to other colleagues and media writers with little comment or acknowledgement. It was not reviewed in the popular press, or in the three medical newspapers. In my discussions with colleagues and our medical organisations, both political and academic, I got little support for my views about the iniquitous and divisive two-tier system and the for-profit hospitals. The Irish Medical Organisation (IMO) appeared to oppose the minister on the issue initially, but chickened-out when it came to a crunch – it was more concerned about the consultants' contract. The Royal College of Physicians showed little interest, despite its responsibility for standards of ethical behaviour and professional practice among its members and fellows. The President of the Royal College of Surgeons was interested and sympathetic, but felt that he could not influence some of his colleagues on the for-profit issue.

The head of the HSE and the chief executive of my own hospital group both gave me a long, sympathetic and detailed interview, but were of course not in a position to make any criticism or comment. I was received by Mary Harney and three senior staff in her department. She listened with patience and courtesy to my views and before the interview ended she asked for clarification on a number of points I had made. Apart from one comment, the three officials remained silent. I left the interview with the distinct impression that the minister had little insight into the vocation and traditions which are an inherent part of a caring profession, and that she was motivated by the principles of economics rather than social justice. Her proposals were too political to allow comment or input by her officials. It was a confirmation that Mammon is still supreme in our Republic despite the sentiments of the 1916 signatories and our politicians' endorsement of these sentiments on the occasion of the Rising's ninetieth anniversary. Were our political masters really sincere in their tributes to our noble dead and their aspirations? Or were they motivated more by vanity, electoral and political considerations?

SIPTU (representing four major trade unions, including the Irish Medical Organisation), in its proposals prepared for the Social Partnership negotiations in 2006, resolved to oppose the privatisation of the health service. However, the matter was not raised by its representatives at the negotiations. When I enquired of one SIPTU official afterwards, I was told that it would be raised at further negotiations in the autumn of that year. I heard nothing further, nor is there evidence that the matter was ever raised. As long as financial considerations were settled and the senior officials of the combined trade unions appeared to have done their job to the satisfaction of their members, such social problems were probably not relevant to their own aspirations.

My views mirrored those of a number of ardent critics of Mary Harney's policies but they, like myself, must feel that money and power will succeed where more informed and vocational issues are thought naïve and quixotic. The best health systems in terms of equity and efficiency are the single-tier compulsory insurance systems found in the Scandinavian countries, and also in France, Germany and Austria.

During my presidency of the IMA I was invited to attend the annual general meeting of the British Medical Association in Kuala Lumpar and Singapore where the medical associations of the commonwealth countries were represented. It was a contentious assembly, because several of the newly-elected commonwealth countries from the Caribbean and elsewhere, on joining the commonwealth group at this meeting, successfully voted South Africa out of the association because of its apartheid policies. This was against the wishes of Britain and the older commonwealth countries, which I supported, but I regretted afterwards that I did not approach the newcomers to modify their rather hostile initiative. It was only later that I realised how Ireland could have considerable influence with the emerging colonial countries and that my intrusion might have had some effect in postponing the expulsion of South Africa. This political intrusion cannot have helped the spirit of the Commonwealth Medical Association.

As a longstanding member of the IMA's executive, I was appointed as the Irish representative on the Union of European Medical Specialists. We were mainly concerned with the standardisation of medical training, practice and specialist registration in the early days of the European Union, all to facilitate the possibility of doctors being permitted to practice in other Member States. My role involved several visits to Europe during the 1970s and underlined the need to brush up my schoolboy French. English had not yet become the *lingua franca* of Europe and we were provided during our meetings with an expensive and cumbersome translating facility with English, French, German and Dutch available but generally mish-mashed in the process. Nowadays all medical meetings in Europe are conducted in English, largely because of the Anglo-American influence in science and world medicine.

I cannot say if our meetings had any worthwhile influence on standardisation or medical practice within the expanding Union. Certainly, few practising doctors or specialists seem to have crossed borders since. Our deliberations were rather tiresome and unreal. Clearly any realistic coming-together of the professions in our different countries needed to overcome the widely differing cultures of medical practice, particularly between the Anglo-Irish and European jurisdictions. On such a visit to Montpellier, that historic and gracious city in Languedoc, I met three or four colleagues who may have had the answer to the paucity of cross-border medical migrations. After my visit to their hospital they entertained me to lunch. It was the usual French lunch, lasting at least two hours and with the jeroboam of *vin de pays* gracing the table. My French was execrable but apparently intelligible enough to allow the following exchange to take place

I said 'Now that Ireland has joined the European Union, *que pensez-vous de la proposition que je travaille ici a Montpellier?* (What do you think of the idea that I come to work in Montpellier?) After a pause, their spokesman said: '*En France nous aimons la touriste et le visiteur mais nous n'aimons pas l'étranger!* (In France we like tourists and visitors but we do not like strangers!)

I decided to stay in Dublin. The only benefit I gained from my essay into the medical politics of Europe was a smattering of French, which I keep alive by listening to the French radio station, France Inter, in my car. I wonder if the country or the Union gained much by our meetings and recommendations. I remained in the IMA until it joined the Medical Union and thus took on the mantle of a trade union. I resigned then but rejoined in 2006 to support the forces against Minister Harney's two-tier system and profit-motivated private hospitals. When the IMA relented on this issue, I resigned again, only to be elected an honorary member. I accepted the honour in the spirit with which it was conferred.

15

THE IRISH CARDIAC SOCIETY

My senior colleague at St Vincent's, Dr Patsy O'Farrell, was a rather gruff and non-communicative individual, almost certainly evidence of an unusual degree of shyness. Nevertheless, he was more progressive than most of his contemporaries. He was president of the College of Physicians in Ireland and of the combined British and Irish Medical Associations; he was the Irish representative at the London-based Medical Defence Union, which acted for most of the Irish doctors. He had a strong interest in cardiology and was a member of the British Cardiac Society from its foundation. Like all his colleagues in these years, he was a general physician with an interest in heart disease, but he was not familiar with the great advances made in cardiac diagnosis immediately after the war, nor did he strike me as being comfortable in dealing with patients.

As evidence of his initiatives, after my arrival at St Vincent's he suggested setting up an Irish Cardiac Society and invited me to act as its honorary secretary. We had the first preliminary meeting in November 1950. About sixteen colleagues from the various Dublin hospitals joined, although few had a specific and none an exclusive interest in heart disease. The Society has since thrived, although its activities in the early years varied from time to time depending largely on the energy and enthusiasm of the prevailing honorary secretary. The purpose of the society was to exchange information about research and progress in cardiology, to hold annual meetings and to advise the health authorities about the needs and standards of cardiology in the hospitals and health service. It was at a meeting of the Cardiac Society in 1965 that the formation of a heart foundation was mooted, and later in the 1960s that the recommendation to have a surgical heart centre in the Mater Hospital was proposed, an important step in developing and rationalising our surgical services.

In early 1951 I suggested to Dr O'Farrell, the founder and first president, that I might approach our cardiological colleagues in Belfast with an invitation to join the society. There was no contact at that time between the physicians in the Republic and the North. With O'Farrell's approval, I wrote to the two senior cardiologists at the Royal Victoria Hospital asking for an interview. This was arranged and I arrived in the hospital one morning while one of them was doing ward rounds. I was kept waiting for an hour and a half. I did not receive the usual courtesy accorded to visiting consultants of attending and taking part in the ward round. Eventually I was invited to meet my host who was sitting in the sister's office surrounded by his nurses and residents. I was immediately asked the purpose of my visit (already known to him) and, on answering, I was humiliated in front of this formidable gathering when, after a long pause, he said, mispronouncing my name, 'Mulcahy, I want you to know that our loyalties here are to London, not to Dublin' – and I was forthwith dismissed! And indeed this was true, for at the time the Belfast physicians were fellows of the Royal College of Physicians in London and had no contact with the College or their colleagues in Dublin.

Despite this rebuttal, the visit was not without its benefits. I was met after the interview by Frank Pantridge, famed later for his cardiac ambulance and his defibrillator, who had recently been appointed as a cardiologist to the Royal Hospital. I also met with Mollie McGeown, another recent appointment to the staff. Both were furious at the treatment I received by their senior colleague and both did everything to comfort me. They became friends of mine, and later I was to meet John Pemberton, the professor of epidemiology at Queen's University, and Peter Froggatt, later to become vice-chancellor of Queen's. All showed a fine degree of political ecumenism which was sadly lacking in the old guard.

Later still I met Michael Scott and his wife Maureen, also a doctor, who were to become lifelong friends with Louise and me. I met a host of other physicians when the Corrigan Club was formed in 1959 at the behest of two colleagues, Ivo Drury of Dublin, and Douglas Montgomery from Belfast. The Corrigan Club was to copper-fasten the coming-together of physicians from both jurisdictions and was to lead to a substantial change in Northern loyalties from London to a partnership between Belfast, Dublin and the rest of Ireland. The club is now in its fifty-first year and is still going strong. Its serial history is summarised by me in every ten-year membership booklet published by the club.

Dominick Corrigan, after whom the Club is named, was an outstanding physician in Dublin in the mid-nineteenth century and was noted for his contributions to cardiac diagnosis and treatment. He was one of a group of physicians who brought eponymous fame to the Dublin school of medicine at that time. He was the first Catholic to be elected President of the Royal College of Physicians in Ireland, then in its one hundred and fiftieth year, and was probably the first Catholic to be appointed a physician to the Queen. The current classical building of the college that graces Kildare Street in the heart of Dublin was built during Corrigan's unusually long tenure as president.

Today the Corrigan Club is thriving with a membership of 120 physicians from all parts of Ireland. My continuing interest in the club, of which I was a founder member, is not only on the professional side but also in the social activities of the group and, perhaps more than any other reason, in the political contribution such contacts have made to North–South reconciliation. There were many other lasting friendships which endured as well as the Scotts and ourselves.

The earlier Northerners were not the only colleagues to ignore the Irish College. Sometime in the 1930s there was a dispute between the physicians in the two Catholic hospitals in Dublin, St Vincent's and the Mater, and the college. As a result, most of the physicians in these two hospitals refused to sit the College examinations. As St Vincent's and the Mater advanced in importance as service and teaching hospitals attached to University College Dublin, the conflict led to increasing embarrassment for the College of Physicians. It was decided to offer fellowships to the difficult colleagues but, to achieve this without appointing honorary fellowships, the rules of the college needed to be bent slightly.

I did not do the examination for the Irish college because I was trained in London and had been admitted a member of the London College. I therefore was included in the list of seven physicians who 'sat' the examination which admitted us as members of the Irish college. After the examination had concluded (during which I was asked only one question – about cigarette smoking and health), I was forthwith admitted as a member and then immediately as a fellow by the president of the college. It was an Irish solution to an Irish solution to an Irish problem, but was none of the worst for that. We were later conferred and I have a nice photo of us posing outside the classical façade of the college in Kildare Street. Unlike their senior colleagues, the physicians in the North are active members of the Irish college and several Northern physicians have been presidents of the college in recent years.

Professor John Pemberton was responsible for organising the All-Ireland Social Medicine Society. John was English and was head of preventive medicine in Queen's University; he once said to me that he could never understand Northern politics. His initiative was a valuable ecumenical contribution to uniting the Irish profession at clinical, research and academic levels. Its first meeting was held in 1968 and it continues to meet every two years in various parts of the island. With our epidemiological interests, I was active in the group in the early days and was joined by Noel Hickey, Ian Graham and others of our research group.

The medical profession, like other professional and sporting bodies, played an important part in bringing about the gathering reconciliation between the North and South. John retired to England and died recently at the age of ninety-four. He was a stalwart member of my profession.

16

THE WORKERS

My professional life was hugely satisfying because of my interest in clinical cardiology and my strict adherence to hands-on bedside and clinical practice, as opposed to the more distant and technical approach practised by latter-day cardiologists. It was the freedom from more technical preoccupations that provided me with the opportunity of maintaining close contact and satisfactory communication with patients and their relatives, and of following a career in clinical research. I had the good fortune to join the ranks of the cardiovascular epidemiologists who did so much at an international level to advance the knowledge and to reduce the impact of the coronary epidemic. My friends abroad added to the pleasure of visits to so many countries worldwide. I was fortunate too in commencing a long-standing research programme into heart disease in my hospital and having the benefit of so many wonderful friends and professional colleagues. Finally, in that way, I have been lucky all my life.

During my time from 1961–1988, I was accompanied as a clinician and researcher by Noel Hickey, except for a gap of a few years in the early 1960s. He played a seminal role as medical director of the Irish Heart Foundation and director of the hospital's department of health promotion. He followed me as professor of preventive cardiology and joined me on the international circuit. He was appointed senior lecturer in the

Department of Epidemiology at University College Dublin. His death six years after my retirement was a serious loss to me personally, to preventive medicine and to his hospital and university.

As a natural-born epidemiologist and as the son of a doctor, he was aware of the importance of maintaining his involvement in clinical medicine. I was always happiest when working with Noel. To him, his Hippocratic obligations extended beyond the sick patient to the community at large. He understood more than anybody the profession's responsibility of promoting good health as well as looking after the sick and the infirm. Noel was too rational, intelligent and spiritual to have been satisfied by such mundane aspirations as material acquisitions and monetary gain. His life was more successful and more productive than most, if we are to measure success in terms of his professional contributions to public health, in terms of serenity of mind and of a philosophical disposition, of his many devoted friends and patients, and of the affection and pride he evoked in his wife and family. He had a devotion to his splendid garden, where he was happiest, and his material demands were limited. It is said that, to be happy all one's life, one should become a gardener. Noel surely was aware of this adage, and of the contribution his garden made to the tranquillity and security of his household and to the interest of his many visitors.

Ian Graham came from Trinity College, Dublin, and Cambridge University to St Vincent's in 1978 and spent five years with us as a senior research fellow with consultant status. He had been my registrar in 1975 and I was fortunate to have him back to supervise our research activities. Apart from his clinical skills, he was a born-investigator with a clear, logical mind. He supervised several research projects with us, including a programme of cardiac rehabilitation sponsored by the European Union. He led an eighteen-month study to identify the efficacy of defibrillation in a hundred successive patients in the hospital who suffered cardiac arrest. He set up a detailed register in the coronary care unit, where audit became an important and necessary feature of our practice.

With the staff of the Irish Heart Foundation and the Mater Hospital, he organised a national cardiac surgery register, which for some time produced annual reports of the outcomes of heart surgeries (but sadly came adrift because of some opposition from surgeons and poor financing). He was later appointed to the Adelaide Hospital, where he continued the same policies of research and inpatient management. He was to make major contributions to heart disease prevention on the international circuit during his distinguished career in the Adelaide and later in Tallaght, and was appointed to chairs in cardiology in the Royal College of Surgeons and in Trinity College.

Leslie Daly of the UCD School of Public Health and Population Sciences was our statistician since 1976 and is still attached to the university and St Vincent's as Professor of Epidemiology and Biomedical Statistics. Lead author of some of our more important research papers, Leslie's interests have spread into many areas of social and medical research. He was preceded in this role by Gilbert McKenzie of Queen's University. The statisticians had all the skills and essential qualities of their arcane trade, including the prima donna trait – without which no statistician is worth his salt. They are the custodians who keep a close eye on our research data and conclusions. Looking back on our history of governance in Ireland and the nation's recent poor record of accountability, those in medical research particularly should remember the adage of our Roman forebears' *quis custodiet ipsos custodes*. Our statisticians served us well.

We were later joined by our polymath, Ronan Conroy, whose position was difficult to classify because of his numerous skills and accomplishments – gifted conversationalist, writer, linguist, statistician, maths and computer genius, instrumentalist and musician. He is now head of the Department of Preventive Medicine in the Royal College of Surgeons in Ireland. Killian Robinson was a prolific writer and innovative member on our staff who eventually left these shores to become a consultant cardiologist in the United States.

We enjoyed the long service of our dietician, Vivian Reid, who maintained her equanimity during the recurring storms surrounding the cholesterol controversy. She retired in February 2009; her predecessor was Aileen Finnegan. Our earliest nurse investigators and comforters, Denise Comerford and Carol Pye, are still serving the hospital and have brought many others into their department and trained them in health promotion. They formed the nucleus of our research team with our longstanding ward sister, Una Leydon, and the nursing staff in the coronary care unit. Like the research staff, the staff nurses in the coronary care unit participated in the counselling of patients about rehabilitation measures and the importance of lifestyle in achieving and maintaining good health.

Geoffrey Bourke and Cecily Kelleher, successive heads of the University School of Public Health, succeeded Noel Hickey as directors of the hospital department, and both provided the link between the hospital and the university. Many others were part of the team for shorter periods, among who were Brian Maurer, David Kilcoyne, Anna Clarke and our three psychologists, Frances Finn, Professor E. F. O'Doherty and Eric Guiry. Déirdre Concannon was our physiotherapist who twice a day kept the patients in coronary care on the move to music and who must accept the credit that no one ever suffered a pulmonary embolus (clot to the lung) or any other obvious complication of confinement to bed. Valerie Feehan looked after our outpatient services for many years and Bob McFarlane played a vital role as head of the lipid laboratory and stickler for reliable methodology.

Our longstanding secretary in the hospital, Nancy Grogan, provided the link between us all. It was she who carried the load of organising our meetings, caring for the finances and supervising the production of most of the 170 peer-reviewed papers which we published, mostly during our thirty-year research period. We could not have functioned without her. My own three private secretaries, Chris O'Doherty, Ann O'Connor, and my amanuensis of nearly forty years, the late Maura Mulcahy, assisted Nancy with publications. Maura was my first cousin, and remained my personal secretary during my entire active medical career. She was my alter ego in every sense, particularly during my absence abroad. I hope she is reading these lines from her celestial abode.

The Sisters of Charity provided at all times for our needs. They were the sole instigators of my new department in 1960 which made our subsequent clinical and epidemiological researches possible. I will forever be grateful to them for their quiet and benign support, and for their understanding. They and our nursing school were the bedrock of the great ethos of St Vincent's Hospital. Since 1834 the Irish Sisters of Charity have played a crucial role in education and in providing many vital social services, long before central and local government adopted such responsibilities.

The Sisters are sadly missed, just as we miss our nurses' teaching school. The St Vincent's Hospital nurses, who like their colleagues trained in other Irish teaching hospitals, are renowned worldwide. The shift of our hospital undergraduate nursing school to the university campus was a retrograde step which has greatly harmed our nursing profession and the ethos of our public teaching hospitals.

17

RETIREMENT
1988–PRESENT

AUSTRALIA

I retired from my two hospitals in October 1988 and was granted a festschrift and a parting reception by the St Vincent's Hospital staff. The festschrift was a collection of some of my publications during my thirty-eight years in the hospital.

After my retirement I went to Australia to attend a world congress on cardiac rehabilitation in Brisbane. I was accompanied by my future wife, Louise Hederman. We stayed in a magnificent casino hotel on the Gold Coast south of Brisbane. The entire ground floor of the hotel was devoted to gambling. At six o'clock every morning, before the heat descended upon us, I went out for a five-mile run. To do so I had to cross the casino floor, where the twenty-four-hour gambling activity was in full swing to the sound of the croupiers and the one-armed bandits. Nobody appeared to take the slightest notice of the scantily clad runner passing through. The Gold Coast, with its profusion of tropical flora, was a magical ambience in which to enjoy the freedom and sensuality of running in the heat.

Travelling from Brisbane to Sydney and from there on to Canberra and Melbourne, we were struck by the remoteness of the continent, its excellent roads extending straight to the horizon and empty of traffic, its vast forests of eucalyptus, and its long distances. Later we visited friends about two hundred miles north of Melbourne. Homesteads were miles apart and, despite the excellent roads, there was a sense of remoteness and isolation everywhere. I was fortunate that I had read *The Fatal Shore* by Robert Hughes before I left Ireland. I knew more than the Australians about their history during the 200 years from the time of James Cook, a circumstance that provided me with some occasions for one-upmanship. We enjoyed a two-week visit to New Zealand, with its 1950s ambience of Anglias and Ford prefects, with its strange trees, with geysers and volcanoes, its clapboard houses and its obvious prosperity. Like Australia, its roads in the North Island, which we travelled extensively, were good but had little traffic. Here too there was a striking sense of remoteness.

A five-month stay in the Austin Hospital in Melbourne, with its tradition of Anglo-Irish medicine, caused little or no culture shock. The roots of the city and its people were clearly laid by the British and Irish. I was invited by Dr Alan Goble to Australia to assist with his cardiac rehabilitation service. His interest as a cardiologist, like mine, was on rehabilitation and secondary prevention. However, my responsibilities were nominal. I did little clinical work in the hospital, spending my time instead learning to type, to use word processors and computers, and to writing a book, *The Long-term Care of the Coronary Patient* (1989). I owed much to Elaine Race, Dr Goble's secretary, for her expert advice which enabled my ageing brain to become quite efficient at word processing and typing.

Both Alan Goble and his colleague, Marion Worcester, received Louise and I with the warmest hospitality, and provided generously for us during our stay in Melbourne. Leaving for home from Perth, I was reminded of the vastness of Australia as we flew for five hours along the deserted west coast of the continent.

After retirement I ceased all hospital and nursing home practice but continued my consultant and medico-legal work at the Charlemont Clinic in Dublin. I retired completely from medical practice in 2005, having spent the previous five years supervising the stress testing facility at the clinic. Retirement has been an active and productive time because of my gathering interest in golf, cycling, running and later walking; my interest in trees, research into the effects of ivy on trees and hedgerows, recent Irish history, the health service, the environment, book reviewing and writing books. I maintained a close contact with my university at the nearby Belfield campus, mainly with its libraries and through my interest in the historical archives where my father's large collection of papers and effects were lodged in 1970 at his behest. The university's six-hundred-acre grounds, with their many fine trees and new plantations and sports fields are availed of by Louise and me for walking, enjoying the outdoor life and meeting some of our neighbours.

The university campus owes much to the pioneering president of the college, Michael Tierney, who was responsible for the move from Earlsfort Terrace. The official move took place in 1960 amid much controversy and friction between students and academic staff; but it was to take another forty-eight years before the last residue of the university left Earlsfort Terrace in 2008!

MY FAMILY

After my retirement, I found myself closer to my children than I ever was during my active professional years. We had three boys followed by three girls. My eldest daughter, Tina, has been living in Strasbourg since 1973 but the other five now live in Dublin or County Wicklow.

After my departure from Lissenfield Richard, our eldest, restored the old cowshed in our grounds and went to live there but continued to provide support for his mother and act as a prop for his five siblings. He kept close to Aileen's two siblings, Miriam O'Donoghue and Richard Hanton, and thus played an important role in preserving the integrity of the extended family. Unlike his two younger brothers, who both went into medicine, he entered the business world and, with his entrepreneurial instincts, he seems to have enjoyed challenge and change. For someone in the business world he has been generous and has maintained high ethical standards, supports various charities and has been particularly close to Louise and myself. He is now well into farming and in organising an Eco village on the borders of Wicklow and Wexford.

I was followed in going to London by my son, David, who spent ten years in the newly-built National Heart Hospital in Chelsea. He subsequently was appointed as a cardiologist to Tallaght Hospital in Dublin. He established a few important initiatives in the heart unit there with his colleagues, particularly in treating acute heart attacks and in preventing sudden death in young people. In referring to David, one of his patients described him as 'a chip off the old block'! His wife, Sharon, prominent in the commercial catering world, is noted for her hospitality and open house in West Wicklow, where they live with their three children.

My youngest son, Hugh, was appointed as a gastroenterologist to St Vincent's Hospital in Dublin. He too trained for some years in London, mainly at St Bartholomew's Hospital. He is part of an international group researching the natural history and management of colorectal cancer and other bowel conditions, along the same lines as my research into coronary disease. His wife and medical colleague, Martha, has established the hub of the extended family in their house in Appian Way. They have three children. It was Hugh who took on the major task of digitising my father's 165 tape recordings. There was no previous tradition of medicine in my family until I joined the medical faculty at UCD. It is naturally a source of pride for me that two of my sons have followed in my footsteps.

After schooling, Tina followed a course of bi-lingual secretarial training and was appointed in 1981 to the staff of the Council of Europe in Strasbourg. She advanced rapidly from this position to the User Support Team, and then, in order, to Chairman of the Staff Committee, Coordinator of User Services in the Directorate of Information Technology, Principal Administrator and Advisor to the Private Office of the Secretary General, and, currently, Executive Director of the European Youth Centre. Phew! She is married to Edmond Perrier, head of medicine in his Strasbourg hospital, Établissement Publique de Santé Alsace de Nord. They have two children. They have made a great contribution to Franco-Hibernian accord at a family and social level.

Both Barbara and Lisa were trained in the College of Marketing and Design and subsequently went into the film business. Barbara, with her exceptional organisational skills and her meticulous attention to detail, became an assistant director responsible for all aspects of film production and planning. Her talents include the ability to control difficult extras with a sharp tongue. She has followed me in her dedication to aerobic exercise and the outdoors and is a welcome walking companion. She is closely involved in the extended family with her devotion to her eleven nieces and nephews.

Lisa became a film director, both in the entertainment and commercial world. Her work includes a full-length film, *Situations Vacant*, which was released in December 2009. She directed many shorter productions, including her memorable *Dan Dan, Dad and Me*, about our three generations. This hour-long film was commissioned by RTÉ in 2000. Its frank and sometimes moving story relating the family history, warts and all, is still talked about. Her partner, Michael Garland, is also in the film business. They have three children, she having acquired twins unexpectedly in her early forties. They live in the uplands above Avoca and the Avonmore River, where they are close to trees and to nature.

TREES

Aileen and I and our six children moved to Lissenfield in Rathmines in 1966. Lissenfield was a commodious house with a garden of more than two acres. It lacked such comforts as central heating and double glazing, and was in a bad state of repair and needed considerable restoration. The garden and outhouses also required considerable attention. By 1966 it had become difficult for my mother to manage. I arranged to buy the lease from the Department of Finance – we had been forty-four years living there – so I exchanged houses with my parents, who were very happy in my home in Temple Villas during their later years, and were devotedly looked after by their housekeeper, Maggie O'Connor. Maggie is still hale and hearty at ninety-five years and remains part of our family.

I marvel, looking back to those years, at the energy I possessed when I undertook, not only to change house with such a large family, but also the task of restoring Lissenfield and its extensive gardens, of adding a new addition to the kitchen area, extensive double glazing, central heating, and rebuilding the outhouses and garden walls. We laid down a tennis court and a new avenue and pathways. It was a monumental task in retrospect.

I planted about fifty specimen trees as part of a modest arboretum in

1966. We already had about twelve mature hardwood trees, including five beeches, a few chestnuts, and a scattering of ash and sycamore, mostly along our avenue. I planted thirty Lombardy poplars along the northern and eastern boundaries of the grounds which grew prodigiously by at least six feet every year. Sadly most of the trees, both recently-planted and mature, are now gone as a developer made the maximum use of the land to build many duplex houses. A number of the young trees in the arboretum were presented by family members and friends because my interest in trees was known. Since then it has been our custom to present a tree as a gift to others, partly because of my interest in encouraging specimen trees but also because I realised that the gift of a tree is always remembered.

My long-term interest in trees was to lead during my retirement to my membership of the committees of the Irish Tree Society and the Irish Tree Council. I represented An Taisce on the latter body. The ITS was established twenty years ago to encourage the growing of specimen trees and to stimulate a public interest in trees. Our four or five outings each year are to arboretums in Ireland and occasionally in the UK or further abroad. Over the years we have visited many of the lesser-known arboretums as well as those frequented by the public. Many of these estates were planted around the same time in Western Europe in the mid-nineteenth century after Douglas, Menzies and other great pioneers and explorers had returned from the North American west coast and other distant lands. Hence many of the trees in the estates were introduced by these pioneers and are of the same vintage. Now, by the new millennium, they are mature or post-mature and are being gradually lost, like our hedgerow trees. It is astonishing how rich Ireland is in gardens and arboretums, many being relics of the old estates and demesnes, and mostly unknown to the public. There are few intact estates in the Republic nowadays, but some remain in Northern Ireland, where they are clearly being threatened by the huge costs of maintenance.

We see a bewildering number of different trees during our outings. I am no expert on tree identification, but we have a few aficionados in the ITS who move about, poring over their books, minutely examining every part of the tree – the leaf, bark, buds, flowers and the shape or habit – and forming little huddles with their peers to discuss some arcane or contentious point about identity or provenance. However, there are other distractions which are more agreeable, such as the company of the many other sociable members of both sexes.

Social life during many of these outings is not neglected and in particular it provides Louise and me with some firm and lasting friends from the North. The Irish Tree Society was one of the many social, professional and recreational bodies which have maintained an important contact between our Northern friends and us in the South while the process of reconciliation moves gradually towards a resolution. I was obliged some years later to retire from my tree committees because of a hearing deficit.

The success of the Irish Tree Society owes much to the enthusiasm and leadership of Thomas Pakenham of Tullynally Castle and the devoted administrative skills of Liam and Maureen O'Flanagan of Castlepollard. Aside from the contribution of the society to the welfare of Irish trees, it will be remembered by posterity by the Millennium oak plantation, which extends over a few hectares that the society established at Tullynally. I was involved for some time in reporting to the society about the Tomnafinnoge forest in Coolattin on the borders of Wicklow and Wexford, the remains of the great 400 hectare Coolattin oak forest which was taken over by developers. It was thanks to the ITS as well as other organisations, to local intervention and to some political influence, that the 60 hectares that were left of the forest were rescued from the claws of the developers.

The widespread interest in trees among our great estates was largely thanks to the encouragement of the Royal Dublin Society, an organisation established in the 18th century in Dublin with the aim of advancing agriculture, industry, arts and science. Before I resigned from the ITS committee in 2007, I had induced the post office authorities to publish four stamps commemorating the ash, the oak, the arbutus and the yew – trees which are native to Ireland.

The sequoias, the great redwoods of the west coast of the United States, can be found scattered around Ireland in ones and twos in our many old estates. The sequoias were first reported by Jk Leonard in 1833 and introduced to Europe by Douglas, Menzies and others after travels to North America in the 19th century. There are many sequoias in the old Irish arboretums but it is doubtful if they will achieve the same size and longevity as those of their native habitat because of our different climate and environment. At the end of my road in Clonskeagh, in the old Roebuck estate, there are nineteen redwoods, all Wellingtonias. They must certainly be the most numerous group of sequoias here. Sadly, two have died recently, two are moribund, and a few others are showing early evidence of deterioration, all from the ravages of honey fungus infestation, an organism which attacks the roots of trees and is, in the circumstances of the closely-scattered sequoias, impossible to control. There are also mature chestnuts, lime and beech trees close-by, which so far appear to be immune to the disease.

I planted about thirty acres of Sitka, Japanese larch, Douglas fir and Scots Pine in west Wicklow in 1974. I had bought about 40 acres of poor agricultural land with a derelict cottage as a family holiday home but it was never restored and lived in because of my subsequent departure from the family. I instead planted most of the land. Despite early difficulties and replantings, the trees thrived with little wind-blow or other damage. There are four plantations in all close to the shore of the Poulaphouca reservoir and facing the magnificent panorama of the King's River Valley. One seven-acre plantation has not been thinned to compare its ultimate development with those which have been thinned. The grants for private planting were modest at that time and we were to wait many more years before newly planted hardwoods earned the generous grants of the EU and the Celtic Tiger.

My modest woodlands qualified me later to join and attend meetings of the Irish Timber Growers Association. Membership of the ITGA provided opportunities to visit the woodlands and forests of Ireland, both north and south, and to meet foresters. It was a time of great interest in forestry in Ireland, which saw a substantial addition to our forests, albeit it from a historically low base. I largely neglected my own woodlands because of my busy professional career but fortunately trees will thrive as long as they have minimum supervision and are not victims of natural disaster, such as fire or a hurricane. In my case I have had few problems.

A special interest has been in the widespread infestation of hedgerow and woodland trees by the common Irish ivy, *hedera helix hibernica*. I published a book on this ubiquitous plant, *For Love of Trees*, in 1996, having researched the subject for twenty years or more and having taken hundreds of photos. I was conscious of the ubiquity of ivy, not only on trees but also on buildings, ruins, hedgerows and every thing capable of supporting and protecting the climber. The common ivy is widespread in Ireland, particularly in the east, southeast, south midlands and west midlands, present elsewhere but less extensive in the northeast and less virile in the west. It grows on trees at a rate of three to four feet every year. It is a climber without branches and flowers while it is climbing but it becomes shrub-like or arboreal once it teaches the top of the structure it is attached to. Once it reaches the higher portions of a tree it leads to loss of leaf cover and of lateral branches and then to the distortion of the tree's natural habit or shape. Once it reaches the canopy it will further destroy the natural shape of the tree and, to most eyes, the tree's aesthetic character. The warm and bright colour of the leafless hardwood tree's bark in the low winter sun is lost. Examination of the roots of a heavily infested tree will confirm that they are heavily entangled by the roots of the ivy, which can be vigorous and extensive, thus depriving the tree of nutrients and water. My observations confirm that every species of tree is vulnerable to ivy's attention.

The serious loss of hedgerow hardwood trees in Ireland in recent years can be attributed to excessive ivy growth as much as to monoculture and the flailing of hedges as part of the REPS scheme and of the mindless activities of some local authorities. The publication of my monograph and a subsequent flier I wrote for the Department of the Environment on the subject gave rise to considerable controversy, but I can claim that, as far as I know, I am the only person in Ireland to have done any research on the natural history of the plant. It is hard to understand those who are indifferent to the aesthetic and destructive effects of excessive growth of ivy on our hedgerow and woodland trees. Indeed, it seems that most people are not aware of the ivy problem and seem to have little interest in the state of our trees.

HISTORY AND BIOGRAPHY

Reading has been my greatest leisure activity except during my busiest clinical and research times. When asked how I have managed to fit so many activities into my life I answer, 'I do not look at television except when a programme of special interest is brought to my attention and I am a scanner of newspaper headlines'. History has been one of my principal reading interests but biographies have had the greatest influence on my life. I have not read fiction for sixty years or more.

During my active clinical and research career I had little time for general reading as I had to keep up with the medical literature. I acquired my first computer, an Apple, in the mid-1990s, after which I adopted the routine habit of writing a review of every book I read. Reviewing is an exercise in writing and in retaining a 'quick-fix' method of remembering the principal contents of each book. A few of these were invited by the *Irish Times* and the medical press but most were for my own archives and for occasionally sharing with other readers.

A few books have been of special interest and influence over my life and career. Harvey Cushing's biography, *Sir William Osler*, was hugely influential in establishing pride in my profession and its ethos, and in guiding my clinical work and my relationship with patients. Rather than being irked by 'difficult patients', I found such encounters challenging and a source of satisfaction when resolved; the more difficult, the more challenging. Osler's essays, including his *Aequenimitas*, could not but move the reader; at one time in my clinical career I used to present my resident doctors with a copy of it.

White's *Heart Disease* was first published in 1931. It was the third edition in 1944 which led me to choose a career in cardiology, despite tempting opportunities to specialise in other areas. In his writings and his famous textbook, White was a leader in educating the profession about heart disease.

The meditations of Marcus Aurelius were my spiritual *vade mecum* and left me without the need to depend on formal religion. From the time I first read the meditations I accepted the stoic philosophy, which I interpreted as being the belief that God was immanent in the world in the form of virtue. The Stoics were an elitist group, virtuous and unworldly. They originated in Greece but were probably most influential in Rome at the time of Christ. They preceded Christianity and I believe the Christian philosophy of virtue and love for our fellow man owes its origin to the Stoics.

The Rights of Man was my political bible. I admired Thomas Paine for his radicalism, his courage and his extraordinary foresight in proposing most of the social services which were revolutionary for his time but which are now an intrinsic part of modern democracies. I admired him too for his stand against privilege and the abuse of power by the few and his support for republicanism and democracy. I wonder what he would think of our democratic system in Ireland, where the executive holds excessive power, where the Dáil and Senate have limited influence and where patronage and corruption are tolerated by government and the people as the norm.

Thomas Robert Malthus was an inspiring and inspired writer on population. His 1798 classic, *An Essay on the Principle of Population*, was my first clue to the disaster that could be the end result of the current explosion in the human population. I first alluded to the threat of over-population in the inaugural Irish Heart Foundation Mulcahy Lecture in 1989. Unfortunately, the world is in complete denial about this issue, a subject I will return to later

I remember 1954 as the year I read Gibbon's *Decline and Fall of the Roman Empire*. It was my first introduction to classical history. It was a reminder of the joys of good writing and good literature.

The Dublin physicians in the Meath and Richmond hospitals during the mid-nineteenth century were well known internationally for their clinical advances and their bedside teaching methods. Previously medical teaching had been of a more academic nature and gave little impetus to the close insight doctors require in dealing with their patients' physical and psychological needs. Several of these Irish physicians published important textbooks on matters dealing with the heart, arteries and the lungs. I developed an interest in the lives and contributions of these nineteenth-century predecessors, and I published seven articles for the Irish and British medical press based on an interpretation of their diagnostic and treatment concepts in the light of modern cardiology. In terms of modern diagnostic and therapeutic cardiology, they were light years behind our current knowledge but, in providing information about the heart and its diseases at the time, they formed a vital link between the complete ignorance of former times and today's wealth of knowledge.

I addressed meetings of the Royal Irish Academy of Medicine, the British Cardiac Society and the Boston Medical Society on these nineteenth-century Irish predecessors. Many doctors have become absorbed in medical history and have devoted their lives to exploring the past. It can be an absorbing subject and can teach us much about our profession; but for me my interest was terminated after a few years. I became fully occupied by coronary disease research and management.

With Oliver McCullen, my ear, nose and throat colleague, I occupied private rooms in the house of William Doolin at 2 Fitzwilliam Square. Doolin was a surgeon at my hospital but was better known as a writer, literary aficionado and editor of our two medical journals in Dublin. He was immensely interested in my historical writings and was of considerable help to me in the early stages of my writings. I recall him saying to me on the day before I gave my first address to the Royal Academy of Medicine in Dublin, 'When you are addressing the meeting speak directly to some person in the back of the hall.' Just as I nervously mounted the podium at the meeting after being introduced by the chairman, the door opened and Doolin appeared and sat at the back of the auditorium! There was no microphone then and it was a lesson I have never forgotten.

Part of my time in retirement was devoted to examining my father's military and political papers. He had been chief of staff of the revolutionary army from March 1918 to January 1922 when the Angle-Irish Treaty was ratified by the Dáil, and he was head of the Free State army during the greater part of the Civil War. For my father and mother these were stirring times; and for my five siblings and me, living in an inner-suburb of Dublin in the 1920s and 1930s, the after-effects of the revolution were never far removed from our lives.

My family background and my parents' influence were to play a large part in my own impulses, ambitions and career. I have taken an active part in recent years in attempting to rehabilitate my father's reputation as a key military and political figure in the 1916–1924 period, between the Rising and his retirement as minister of defence at the time of the Army Mutiny in March 1924. His biography, *Portrait of a Revolutionary: General Richard Mulcahy and the making of the Irish Free State*, was published by Maryann G. Valiulis in 1992. She describes him as the 'forgotten hero', which indeed had an element of truth and which could be attributed to his modesty and self-effacement, and his refusal to discuss his controversial early career during his active life and his refusal to release his extensive papers until the year of his death. His military reputation was diminished by the passage of time, and by a long and mundane political career spent mostly in opposition, after the revolutionary period, having been overshadowed by the gathering cult of Michael Collins.

During his active career he eschewed public discussion about his role and the events of these stirring times, but after retirement he threw himself with characteristic energy into recording his memoirs. I acted as his literary executor and arranged facilities for him to archive his extensive papers, to record on tape his experiences during the revolution and many of his conversations with colleagues, historians and his family. My own family memoir, *Richard Mulcahy: a Family Memoir*, published in 1999, describes aspects of his life and career and the lives of my mother and her siblings, some of whom were also prominent during the revolutionary period. I published a biography of my father in June 2009, entitled *My Father, the General* (Liberties Press).

THE IRISH LANGUAGE

During more than eighty years of self rule we have failed to restore our beautiful and ancient language to its proper place in our lives – this despite much investment in time, education and money, and in abundant lip service. Failure in this regard can be traced to unwise policies and the unwillingness of the great majority to restore the language as part of our heritage. My own experience of Irish is a parable of what has happened in the language movement. My father was an excellent self-taught Irish speaker. After the Treaty he was instrumental in establishing Irish-speaking schools; he put his six children through Irish-language primary and secondary schools. When young we had my father to share the language with and at all times had a governess from the Gaeltacht to supervise our studies and to speak the language in the home. As a child, my siblings and I spoke good, if somewhat childish, or *tinteán*, Irish. Of course there was much English too as neither my mother nor the kitchen staff spoke Irish.

I joined the medical faculty in UCD in September 1939, where my new friends had all been to English-speaking schools. All had passed Irish in the leaving certificate, but few if any could speak the language, nor did they have any commitment to its survival. From my entry to the university I hardly spoke another word of Irish until I retired from my hospital in 1988, and by then I had forgotten the language. It was after my retirement that I felt an increasing regret that I had forsaken the language and that I had never spoken Irish to my father after leaving school. He savoured the language and would have welcomed using it at any opportunity – but was too modest and private a person to insist on speaking it to us after our departure from the home. So it was only then that I began to appreciate the beauty and uniqueness of the Irish I knew as a child and had learned during my many years' holidays in the Kerry Gaeltacht, close to Daingean Uí Chúise. Munster Irish is in my opinion the richest in its idiom, expression and in its resonance.

My total neglect of Irish after leaving home was shared by my five siblings. Our experience reflects the situation which currently exists, where those children who attend our excellent Gaelscoileanna return to their homes and communities where they have little opportunity to speak the language in the English-speaking environment and few would be found to speak the language as a vehicle of normal conversation outside their schools.

Other problems have had a deleterious effect on the language movement. The compulsory tradition and the *deóntas*, or 'grant', to the people of the Gaeltacht areas has brought the language into disrepute, and it has not been helped by a Parliament which is primarily English-speaking. My experience is that when politicians speak in Irish it is a form of lip service which is dished out to confirm the speaker's patriotism and to conform to political correctness. This does more harm than good to the language. Few public representatives have fluent Irish, a reflection of the lack of commitment to our language by our politicians and the great majority of the Irish people.

Without love for the language and a deep respect for our Gaelic culture, the revival of the language will remain in the doldrums, as indeed it has done in the eighty-eight years of independence. With English becoming the lingua franca of this globalised world, it is unlikely that Irish will ever become an important, functional language. But there are reasons why we should support a revival. We need to have a vibrant Irish language to maintain our cultural heritage just as we need English as a spoken language with its worldwide use, rich literature and huge lexicon of scientific words. We need a new blend of pride and self-confidence and a strong sense of independence if we are to restore the Irish language to its proper place in the day-to-day affairs of Ireland. The globalisation of English should not prevent the Irish and other nations from retaining their native tongues.

I have been relearning the language since I retired, admittedly in slow stages. Radio na Gaeltachta has been a great help while driving; I can now speak Irish and think in the language, but I am limited by loss of idiom and in learning *na focail nua*, the very many words of a modern, multinational and progressive society which are so different from the everyday conversation of my childhood. I still require a little courage to speak Irish on social occasions, in my golf club and when I meet strangers and patients.

I maintain my tourist French by listening to France Inter on the long wave in my car; I may finish my days mumbling in three different tongues. Indeed with the educational facilities available to us nowadays, with the leisure at hand and the globalisation of the world, it would be a desirable national objective if we were all trilingual with Irish, English and French, German or Spanish.

EXERCISE

Since I stopped running in 1994, I have continued my regular aerobic exercise in the form of walking, cycling and playing golf, and an early-morning callisthenic programme. Much of the decrepitude we see in the elderly is the result of minimal use of the joints, muscles and ligaments – the classic case of 'if you don't use it, you'll lose it'. The avoidance of injury and accident, so important in the elderly, is another benefit of flexibility to counteract our slower reflexes.

Walking should be the mainstay of the active older person. It is an excellent means of maintaining fitness and is both enjoyable and addictive if we persist with it. I try to walk in pleasant surroundings, away from traffic if possible and safe from predators, both human and otherwise. On a windy day, I walk on the leeward side of hedges, buildings and walls. While I enjoy walking with Louise or Barbara, walking alone can be contemplative and provides an opportunity for mental planning when I am writing. And in balance with my years of squash, running and strenuous aerobic exercise, I learnt to achieve transcendental meditation through the hands of my long-standing masseuse, Eileen Fitzsimons.

My wife Louise has been successful in organising chair exercises for several groups of retired people based on the EXTEND programme. After her retirement as a nursing sister from St Vincent's Hospital, she trained in the EXTEND method. Music and other entertainment add greatly to their popularity; it is an excellent source of physical and psychological support to the elderly and is greatly enjoyed by her clients. Originally derived from the League of Health programme, EXTEND owes its origin in Ireland to the inspiration of Isolde McCullough. In the last few years, Louise has been very active in encouraging and promoting EXTEND as the PRO of its committee.

When I went from being a couch potato to a life of strenuous aerobic exercise in my thirties, I did not realise that it takes time and regular, graduated practice to acquire a training effect and thus to achieve an optimum aerobic effect. Hence, I was discouraged initially and thought I was not capable of strenuous running or playing squash. However, with guidance I learned to be patient in the early stages and spent six months or more of graduated exercise before I achieved a degree of fitness to be able to jog or run four or five miles.

Cycling continues to be a useful, enjoyable and practical form of exercise. Although cycling as an easy form of commuting has been seriously neglected by successive governments and local authorities, we are fortunate in Dublin to have many cycle pathways, making it a practical means of getting about. It is also cheap and environmentally friendly. It is safe if one is mindful of the rules of the road: about 80 percent of all bike accidents are caused by the cyclist themselves through carelessness and failure to follow these rules. Cycling is also suitable for older people as long as one's coordination is reasonably normal and when done on suitable safe cycle tracks or roads. I use a fairly light thirty-year-old semi-racing bike which remains in good condition thanks to a re-haul every five years or so. I have also taken advantage of the modern clothing and equipment which permits me to cycle in bad weather and to carry a limited amount of possessions. The widespread cycle tracks around our suburb and the contiguous UCD campus of six hundred acres are a fine resource. There must surely be a huge future for the bicycle as we face serious energy problems in the future.

Despite the decreasing stamina and the slow attrition of strength as I approach my tenth decade, maintaining an aerobic exercise programme will prolong my health and independence, and my psychological wellbeing, confidence and contact with the environment and people. The physically active and physically fit person of seventy-five years will have the same heart, lung and musculo-skeletal function as the person of fifty-five to sixty years who is sedentary. The active person retains his or her muscle strength, bone density, joint mobility and flexibility to a much greater degree than the sedentary.

My longstanding dedication to aerobic exercise as a means of retaining physical fitness, with its advantages of health, stress management and social cohesion, did not change with my retirement. My experience of rowing in university and cycling was followed by a sedentary period of seventeen years, with golf and its dedication to the nineteenth hole as my main sporting and social interest. Thanks to a heavy fall of snow which eliminated golf for a few weeks in 1969, I was introduced to squash and thus to salvation. From my thirty-seventh year I became addicted to active and strenuous exercise on the squash court, followed later by running, including marathons as I turned sixty. After retirement at the age of sixty-six, I continued to run about five days a week, usually for a distance of five to seven miles until at the age of seventy-two I was obliged to have a hip replacement. While the hip replacement was an immediate success and after sixteen years is functionally as good as new, I did not return to running after the operation. Instead I became an active and brisk walker and increased my cycling and golf. I have continued to be active in these areas despite the natural limitations of stamina and strength associated with gathering years.

I am writing these memoirs during my eighty-eighth year. I now take at least one day a week without any formal activity. This is almost invariably a Monday as I walk the eighteen holes of Portmarnock every Tuesday. The day's rest beforehand is essential so that I can exercise without being conscious of the limitations of my age. I can strive along the fairway or rough as well as my younger partners. One must find a balance between rest and exercise, but having established an appropriate balance it is possible to enjoy a satisfying degree of activity without distress or fatigue at any age. Keeping the legs strong is the secret of avoiding early disability and decrepitude. This is why regular walking, cycling and using a bicycle ergometer in the gym or home are so essential.

I have been a longstanding member of Milltown and Portmarnock golf clubs. My parents joined Milltown in 1927 and Pádraig, Elisabet and I joined in the late 1930s. We three were prominent members of the club. Padraig was captain in 1964, held the amateur course record for several years and was later its president and trustee. His wife, Margaret, was lady captain, and deservedly so because of her immaculate swing, her low handicap and her support for the club. Elisabet was lady captain in 1973 and was well known for her golf and bridge skills. I was captain in 1954 but my golf was neglected during my busy years in hospital and my later greater commitment to squash and running.

Despite my neglect of the game, I found golf a fascinating mental challenge because of the need to overcome the element of fear during that moment just as one is about to strike the ball. Unfortunately, the fear element tends to increase as one gets older. My only regret about golf is that such a time-consuming pursuit might have been better spent hill walking or in some other leisure activity bringing us closer to nature.

In recent years I have been diligent in doing callisthenic exercises on rising every morning, after a facial douche of cold water to wake myself up. These exercises are aimed at maintaining flexibility and function and should be preceded and followed by stretching exercises and taking deep breaths. They are not time consuming – taking perhaps about seven or eight minutes – and they can be combined with meditation in those who are so inclined. They are particularly appropriate for those of us who are approaching our later years.

Fifty years of very active aerobic exercise has had a huge influence on my health, my confidence and self-esteem, and my ability to cope with the pressures and occasional frustrations of a busy professional and social life. There is consistent evidence from population studies that a life of aerobic exercise is beneficial in reducing the risk of many chronic conditions, including heart disease, stroke, cancer and Alzheimer's. Exercising the brain is also effective in postponing the cognitive aspects of ageing and here there is evidence from basic research that the vital cells and communicating structures, the dendrites, in the brain are best maintained in those who are most mentally active. This is not surprising, and simply reflects the same benefits of exercise on the muscle fibres and the ligaments, tendons and bones of the body.

In my 159-page paperback, *Improving with Age*, published in 2003, I refer to the influence of aerobic exercise in contributing to heath, longevity, independence and hopefully to a shorter period of disability before one departs from this life. I travelled abroad about ten or twelve times a year as part of my medical research activities or as a representative of the Irish Medical Association on European committees to implement the mutual recognition of medical training and degrees in six EEC countries. I found running to be of huge benefit during my travels. I would set out from the hotel in the early morning before meetings commenced or after the meetings had finished. I might otherwise have been tempted to find myself not getting up with the sun or in the bar more often than was good for me.

Running in strange cities abroad was a wonderful experience. I have a good sense of direction, and could do a five-mile run anywhere without fear of getting lost. Running is an excellent antidote to the boredom which can sometimes accompany professional travel. It allowed me to see many places which I would not have seen had I been cooped up for the length of my stays in a conference hotel.

A few of my colleagues, both men and women, had a similar interest in running, and when they joined me it added enjoyable and intimate companionship that was not found so easily in the conference room. It was a time when my marriage had ended and I was emotionally deprived of the company and the intimacy of a close confidante and companion. I found such comfort in the company of some of my female colleagues who were runners and not infrequently in need of the same social and emotional support as myself. Meetings abroad generally required two or three days, but not infrequently I would stay on for another day in hotels or cities I particularly enjoyed.

I have a large Mercator projection map hanging in my study with coloured pins marking every place I have run in the world, from Tromso in the Arctic to Manila in the Philippines, from Boston in the United States to Wellington in New Zealand, and from Moscow in Russia to San Diego in California. I have run in Hyde Park, Kensington Gardens and

Regents Park in London, the Bois de Boulogne and the Bois de Vincennes in Paris, Central Park in New York and the great Chapultepec Park in the centre of the City – and felt breathless at the latter's elevation of more than two thousand metres. My most memorable run was from Fisherman's Wharf in San Francisco to the Golden Gate Bridge, across to Sausalito and back to San Francisco Park, a distance of nine miles, to be met by and receive the hospitality of an old colleague, Coleman Ryan, who is a cardiologist in that great city. He had spent a year as my registrar during his training at St Vincent's Hospital in Dublin.

I always faced oncoming traffic when running. This is doubly important when abroad, as it is easy to forget that traffic keeps to the right in many other countries. I tried to remember that runners are injured or die on the road more often from being run down than from any other cause, and that such events are more likely to occur at night. In one American study, half of the fifty runners reported killed were running at night. The use of reflective clothing at dusk or night is crucial. I also used to carry a short, stout stick in case of encountering unfriendly dogs; I slowed to a walk in their presence, as they are less likely to be excited by the familiar walker than by the less familiar jogger or runner.

There are excellent opportunities for running when travelling around Ireland and Britain. The quiet roads and hill tracks of Wicklow, the towpaths along our canals, the many beautiful and tranquil places in the west of Ireland, and the widespread system of pathways and walking routes in most parts of Britain provide endless opportunities for walkers and runners. Unfortunately, Ireland is the only country in Europe where many farmers are opposed to public trespass and where walking and running in the countryside is partly restricted. This is a recent trend in Ireland and to be greatly deplored. Our forebears sought the return of the great estates in the late-nineteenth and early-twentieth centuries to the Irish people. The land is held in trust by the farmers but it belongs to the people of Ireland and, ironically, it appears that 80 percent or more of Irish farmers' incomes are derived from grants from our government and the European Union.

I recall a stay in a splendid hotel in Anacapri at the peak of the Italian island of Capri where I was attending a seminar in honour of Ancel Keys, the American physiologist and one of the great pioneers of research into the causes of heart disease. Every evening after the afternoon session, Peter Schnorr, from Copenhagen, and a friend from Norway would join me in running the five kilometres from the hotel downhill to the Blue Lagoon. We divested ourselves of our clothes – we wore swimming trunks under our shorts – dove into the sea from the rocks and swam into the Blue Lagoon through its narrow entrance, despite the protests of the boatmen who wished to solicit our patronage. I had never realised that blue could be so blue. The swim was followed by a glass of beer in the adjoining bar; then, in the cool of the evening, we ran up the five steep kilometres back to our hotel for dinner. Such moments added great enjoyment, bordering on euphoria, and a great sense of fulfilment to my many trips abroad.

AGEING

In recent years I have noticed the onset of certain limitations which are all part of the functional attrition associated with ageing. I am intrigued by these changes. Many of these tend to fluctuate in the sense that they may at first appear rather unexpectedly, vary in intensity from time to time, and not infrequently resolve themselves only to reappear, sometimes many months later.

For example, dryness of the mouth occurs in bed because of reduced saliva production, and dry eyes when I read a book or paper close to a reading lamp. A few segments of an orange are effective during the night to stimulate the salivary glands, and dry eyes are relieved immediately by appropriate saline eye drops which are freely available in pharmacies today. Sleep may be difficult and can be worsened by eating late, by drinking alcohol and caffeine-containing drinks. A mild sedative on going to bed is a great help; it does not have any after-effects, it leads to quick and reasonably profound sleep, and the current small dose remains effective. I sleep less and tend to dream more, particularly during early waking, the so-called REM stage of sleep. Dreaming time can be quite prolonged, or at least appears to be so. Dreams are greatly varied in their content, with elements of frustration and paranoia predominating. I tend to get up early, sometimes as early as six o'clock, and dowse my face several times in cold water or drink a cup of hot water or very weak tea. In this way the sometimes disturbing reality of the dream quickly fades. On returning to bed, I may have a brief period of natural sleep free from dreaming. Regular bedtime would help sleep and possibly reduce dreaming, but this is a counsel of perfection I do not always follow.

Appetite has diminished, as indeed has the tolerance for alcohol.

Food intolerance becomes more frequent and the culprit foods can usually be identified by trial and error. The high-fibre foods, such as muesli, raw vegetables and crudités, are particularly prone to lead to indigestion and flatus. A more recent intolerance of wine, particularly red, causes quite severe leg cramps and may find me hopping around the bedroom in the middle of the night. Cramps are more likely to occur in cold weather and after strenuous exercise, particularly when I try to keep up with Louise.

My right ear has become seriously deaf over the past twenty years. I'm left with a relatively normal left ear but I have become increasingly disabled by lack of clarity, a problem during ordinary domestic and social conversation. I was obliged to resign from the committees of the Irish Tree Society and the Irish Tree Council because of my inability to follow conversations, and particularly that of the soft-spoken women members. After years of putting the problem on the long finger, I finally took my hearing seriously. I acquired a very flimsy (and expensive) aid for my left ear which helped considerably in one-to-one or small group conversations. I hope to acquire the loop facility provided by cinemas, churches, theatres and on television which helps to overcome the hearing deficit. Those with good hearing, including my nearest and dearest, need to be encouraged to speak clearly to avoid misunderstanding and unwelcome irritation.

Sensitivity to cold is another increasing problem. I need to keep warm in the house and yet also to reduce our need for central heating. Thermal underwear, a short scarf, a house cap and an extra pullover in the house are helpful. In the winter I wear my old tweed suits. Our future lifestyle must surely depend on warm clothing and insulation if we are to reduce our CO_2 emissions.

It is inevitable that sexual activity, so important in a loving relationship, is greatly diminished as we age, although the introduction of the erection-enhancing drugs does add to improved sexual function, if such an issue were to persist into later life.

Like all those with normal vision, I have needed increasingly strong glasses for reading from the age of about fifty years. I eventually needed bifocals to improve fine definition of distant objects, which are useful for television, theatre and cinema, but they are unnecessary for driving or for other outdoor activities. I have my vision checked every two years to ensure that there are no changes occurring, such as increasing pressure within the eyes, which might damage the retinal cells and lead to further impairment of vision.

I am now approaching my eighty-ninth year. My hip operation remains an outstanding success. About eight years ago I suffered a rupture of a quadriceps tendon in my knee in America, which was repaired the following day and which has caused me no further trouble. The young surgeon said, 'It will be better than ever'! As far as I could judge, it was. I also have arthritis of my left shoulder, which required keyhole surgery, but otherwise I have been well and very active. But as we get older we tend to get arthritis in other joints. In particular, the shoulder joint, the hands and the fingers can be troublesome. I've had chronic long-standing discomfort in the first carpo-phalangeal joints (the joint at the base of each thumb) of my hands for the past seven years or more. The discomfort has increased slowly over the years but one can learn to live with such discomfort and suppress the pain except when one thinks about it.

Perhaps the management of pain almost exclusively by the use of drugs is not the only approach. There is no doubt that there is a psychological approach to pain management that can reduce or eliminate the need for drugs. I take a paracetemol once in a while, but I'm still not sure whether it actually provides pain relief or whether it is a psychological or placebo effect. Perhaps both elements are important. Of course, certain painful conditions, such as a toothache, cannot be dealt with by such psychological means.

If there is a reasonable alternative, surgery should be avoided at all costs in older people. With appropriate physiotherapy and exercises, and a constructive and optimistic attitude to one's symptom it is vest to avoid surgery and its longer recovery required by the older person. Adding to arthritis and cramps, generalised pains and aches in various parts of the body are non-specific symptoms in an ageing frame. But if none of these are functionally important, I ignore them.

Added to normal hygiene, parts of the skin may benefit by the regular application of a routine skin lotion such as Nivea cream and Intensive Care. This may reduce a tendency to itchiness which is more prone in older skin; but itchiness is best controlled by ignoring it, although an occasional scratch from one's spouse can by very welcome!

Hair loss, both on the body and head, is inevitable as we grow older. I was not conscious of this until about twenty years ago when I was suddenly struck by acute hair loss on the head and to a lesser extent on the body. The diagnosis of alopecia was obvious. However, after a period of six months there was a substantial regrowth, followed about five years later by a similar but less dramatic loss. Since then what was left has remained. It has caused me no concern. I do not need to comb my remaining locks but, in cold weather and while we are attempting to conserve the heating oil, I wear a small scarf and a hat. The day of the house cap may be upon us soon and we may need to unearth granddad's long johns and night shirt.

I have been a regular but moderate consumer of alcohol all my adult life. I have been fortunate that one too many brings on a bout of depression in me which is accompanied by a temporary aversion to drink. An excess also causes a sense of guilt induced by my sensitivity to damaging my health and my physical and mental functions. On the other hand, a regular drink in the evening before supper with one's wife contributes to the same sense of cohesion which was associated with the shared cigarette in former days, and a pint of Guinness after a round of golf is a fitting end to a pleasant day. If you win your match it enhances your self-esteem; if you lose, it is a welcome consolation. An occasional hot whiskey at night on retiring can relieve the discomfort of the common cold or influenza. It provides a little euphoria and perhaps an earlier recovery. Whiskey does not interfere with immediate sleep but tends to have a delayed stimulant effect leading to early waking and insomnia.

During my clinical days when dealing with the elderly, I found that the single commonest source of anxiety among them is concern about loss of memory and the fear of dementia such as Alzheimer's. Most of the worries about dementia are groundless. There is no doubt that as we get to the eighth or ninth decade of our lives our ability to acquire new information declines. This is best illustrated by my own experience. I was always interested in the subject of memory and did not believe that memory was impaired until late in one's life. When I retired from hospital practice at the age of 66 years, I was still running and I decided to test my memory by learning some of Yeats's poems. These included about twenty in all, including such long ones as 'Ben Bulben' and 'Easter 1916'. I found learning poetry a means of relieving the boredom of long-distance running. At this juncture I had little difficulty in learning the poems.

However, in my eighty-eighth year I am finding it almost impossible to learn new poetry, without constant reinforcement by rereading the text. Obviously, I have largely lost the ability to retain new information of a complex nature. But I have not lost my memory for past or recent events and I am probably as good as ever at doing the simplex crossword in the *Irish Times*. There is compelling evidence from international research that using the brain and exercising the memory is effective in preserving cognitive function, just as active aerobic exercise benefits physical function

Like many others much younger than I, I find it difficult to remember names of people, particularly when I encounter them suddenly and unexpectedly; but the problems here are complex and related as much to the frenetic lives we are living nowadays rather than to any organic change in brain function. I may find it difficult to remember the name of a flower, tree or shrub, but I am aware that the word is lying there in the recesses of my brain and that it will be retrieved eventually if I distract my attention to some other subject. I would attribute this problem in transient loss of memory to the more sluggish movement of the impulses along the neural pathways of the brain.

The most common complaint among anxious patients has to do with loss of attention rather than loss of memory. And this is not confined to the elderly. We get home in the evening; our minds are occupied by God knows what; we bang the hall door, throw the keys down as we are changing or moving about, but, ominously, we fail to register where we threw the keys. We cannot find them an hour or two later when, already late, we are rushing out to a meeting or concert. The house is thrown into turmoil and when the keys are found, your wife shouts after you as you rush out the door 'will you for God's sake go to your GP and get your head tested!' Thanks again to our frenetic lives and our frenetic society we suffer from varying degrees of inattention. After all, it is difficult to think of ten things at the same time! Inattention has nothing to do with organic memory loss. It has to do with failure to record what we are doing. It has to do with lack of discipline, with the chaos in our lives. Carry a spare car key in your wallet. (And don't forget a spare pair of glasses in the glove department of your car and a spare battery for your hearing aid). Yes, I am talking to myself.

Perhaps the most interesting and constructive aspect of ageing is one's attitude. We hear so often of the serenity of old age, greatly to be desired but seldom achieved. I must confess that I have not encountered many serene old people. Nevertheless, an aspiration to remain serene is very important and is a worthwhile objective. It is important to remain optimistic and to remind ourselves of the many consolations we have had in our lives.

It is inevitable that we think of death more frequently than young or middle aged people do. We should have no fear of death; instead we should have a curiosity about it and be philosophical about its inevitability. I do not believe in the next world, being satisfied that religion was invented to reconcile us to the dilemma of our mortality. My spirituality is based on the Greek philosophy of the Stoics whose secular concept of God is virtue, all powerful and immanent. I have passed on my family genes. What more do I want? The world will get on without me as it did for many millennia in the past. I continue to have an optimistic state of mind, as I remain active both mentally and physically, as I continue to take part in family and social life, and as I remain independent.

We can enjoy old age just as much as younger people enjoy youth. Maintaining outgoing interests is preferable to being preoccupied with problems and adversities, present and past. Recently, after two months of rain and a bitter north wind, I walked from my clinic through St Stephen's Green and into Grafton Street on one of our first warm sunny mornings in early April. I was struck by the handsome youths and women I passed and I had a brief moment of envy and regret for my own passing youth and for my former vitality. But my negative mood passed quickly as I quickened my pace and as I thanked God for my own good health and good fortune during my life.

More than anything else, the life which I currently enjoy has been due to my remaining as active as I can physically and mentally, within the limits of the ageing process, and by maintaining a strong interest in the world around me. Mental activity is encouraged by reading, becoming a radio buff, solving problems such as the crossword and Sudoku, continuing hobbies and by keeping in contact with family and my surviving friends. I still attend some social functions, meetings and concerts, although I now meet few of my contemporaries and the interests of younger generations are different from mine. We elderly are aware of the kind but slightly patronising attitude of younger colleagues and acquaintances, frequently provided by the introductory greeting, 'You're looking great'. It is necessary to maintain a normal approach and a sense of humour, and to avoid falling into the trap of boasting about one's age!

Far too many older people interpret the symptoms of ageing as being abnormal and will have recourse to their doctor or to some other health professional. We should avoid finding ourselves unnecessarily on the medical treadmill. Too many drugs are being prescribed, particularly for older people, and too often patients with simple clinical problems are sent for 'routine' investigations which can lead to unnecessary prolongation of medicalisation and to the misinterpretation of normal ageing changes. Medical practice has become too intrusive in people's lives, particularly in relation to non-acute and relatively unimportant complaints. In a recent health questionnaire submitted to nineteen retired priests who were being offered an appropriate exercise programme, all were found to be on prescribed drugs and most were on two or more. It did not surprise me, because of the medical profession's involvement in the worldwide drug culture. What is happening in Ireland reflects the same or worse within the European Union. The need to avoid the unnecessary use of drugs cannot be over-stressed if we are to lead natural and independent lives during our later years.

These can be golden years and can be enhanced by retaining a creative interest in affairs and people, and by having a curiosity, and not a dread, about death. For the very old and the chronic sick and disabled, death must be a gift from God.

18

A WORLD IN DENIAL

My first stirrings of interest in the environment came with the reading of Paul R. Ehrlich's book, *The Population Bomb*, in 1960. It stimulated a concern which led the United States and other countries to support birth control, and family planning in some high fertility developing countries. However, Ehrlich's book evoked strong opposition from the Roman Catholic Church and other religious and fundamentalist groups. Other writers before and after Ehrlich were to refer to the threat of excess human population but there was little response worldwide to their warnings. Thanks to such opposition, much of Ehrlich's influence was to diminish and there is now almost a conspiracy of silence on the subject of human population.

It was shortly afterwards that I read *The Principle of Population*, by Robert Malthus, first published in 1798. I was fascinated by the natural history of species population and control as conceived by him. No work, apart from Darwin's The Origin of Species received so much attention, both approbation and criticism. His concept of population science is still the subject of controversy but to my mind his views are based on sound judgement and his predictions are coming to pass today as our population soars to towards 7 billion; this from a population of just over 3 billion when Ehrlich published his insightful book in 1960.

The substance of Malthus's writings was based on his belief that every animal species, including man, will increase in numbers by geometric progression every generation if they exist in an optimum milieu where checks on survival do not exist. Geometric progression implies doubling in numbers every generation (1, 2, 4, 8, 16 etc). An optimum milieu exists for humans in the absence of civil strife, war and the former epidemic diseases, and provided that there is adequate nutrition for the entire population. These ideal circumstances are consistent with optimum survival and they exist today because of the triumph over the calamitous and devastating contagious diseases of former times, the reduction in famine because of the better production and distribution of food, and the relatively few deaths in war in relation to the total population.

But while the population continues to increase at an estimated 80 million a year, food production will inevitably be limited by lack of resources and significant environmental changes. Malthus gave a few example of such population increases in his first book in 1798 and in his last book published in 1830, he reported that the Irish population had increased from about one million at the end of the seventeenth century to 6.5 million by 1820, no doubt the result of the plentiful potato and a rural population free from the more devastating contagious diseases seen in urban areas.

My concern about human population increase was first expressed when I was invited to give the inaugural Irish Heart Foundation Mulcahy lecture in April 1989, which was subsequently published in the *Irish Journal of Medical Science*. I was speaking about the decline in coronary disease mortality which had begun in the early 1970s. However, I finished my lecture on the note that, while we could feel some satisfaction about the outlook for heart disease control, a much greater long-term problem facing humanity was the inexorable rise in human population. My apparently irrelevant and unexpected reference to population at this juncture was received by a puzzled audience.

I wrote to the Irish Episcopal Council, the Synod of the Church of Ireland, and Archbishop Murphy O'Connor of the Westminster diocese on the Christian churches' need for a new spiritual dimension to protect the environment and to control human fertility. The Christian churches do little to remind the faithful about the importance of the environment and its vital role in the wellbeing of future generations. The wellbeing of the planet is an integral part of Creation, and the care of it is as much a part of our obligation to God as following the other Christian virtue. I can imagine no greater mortal sin than the threat modern society poses to future generations and to Nature.

I need hardly say that I received no reply to my proposals, except for a simple acknowledgement from the Synod. The following year I wrote again to the bishops and the Synod but without a response. Of course in writing to the Catholic bishops I was incredibly naïve and quixotic, but I had to get the impulse off my chest. I have written several letters to the newspapers on population, a few of which have been published, and several to the medical press. They rarely evoked a response.

In 2009 I was invited to join the England-based Optimum Population Trust as a life member. The OPT is a viable and increasingly influential organisation in the UK but it has a long way to go before it influences the politicians and the public on the need for population control. England is now the most densely populated country in Europe. With the late Dr Paddy Hilary, I was invited to be a patron of the Irish Doctors' Environmental Association soon after its foundation. I do not think IDEA has been radical enough in its policies. I think we should be campaigning on the fundamental causes leading to global warming and environmental degradation, unpopular our policies may be to a complacent, acquisitive and denying public.

There is a serious imbalance between humanity and Nature. If we are to save the planet and to ensure a future for our children we need to adopt stronger measures than changing our light bulbs or swapping CO_2 quotas. We need to eliminate waste and we need a change in our greedy and materialistic culture, a drastic reduction in energy usage, a sacred respect for all other species and, most of all, a return to community living and to reduced human fertility. The loss of species should warn us of our own vulnerability; and the loss of trees is crucial. Jared Diamond, in his book, *Collapse: How Societies Choose to Fail or to Survive*, shows how we cannot survive without our trees and forests. European farmland bird populations are down by 50 percent since 1980; amphibian species are in serious decline worldwide, as are many of the world's plants. The decline of species is largely ignored because it seems so gradual and insignificant, but it is very real and decline in most cases is accelerating. Before we realise it, many species will be gone and, indeed, many have gone already. The secretary general of the United Nations, Ban Ki-moon, has warned that species decline has serious consequences for us all.

I am reminded of a parable. One of my grandsons in years to come is asked by his boy of seven years who was holding a ceramic model of a blackbird in his hand. 'Dad, is it true they used to fly through the air?' 'Yes, the blackbird and most other birds used to fly in our garden and all over the world when I was young.' The boy paused in thought and wonder, and then looked up and said 'Dad, why are you crying?'

I believe it is an urgent matter that, to save the earth as we found it and to protect future generations and the natural world, we need urgent and effective action to counteract the damage to our planet. But nothing can be done without the initiative and intervention of our politicians; and yet there is little evidence that our politicians or those of other nations have the will or the intention to take effective measures to reverse current trends. All we need do is look at the failures of Copenhagen. Our politicians are powerless as long as they are motivated by electoral issues, by big business and by their commitment to globalisation. They have let us down badly. And such action as we are taking in Ireland, such as building incinerators is ultimately futile and is simply treating symptoms – but not causes.

When I was a teenager in the mid- and late 1930s, we were an extended family living in a largely suburban community and close to our cousins, neighbours and friends. We had no car, but used our legs, the bicycle and public transport. We rarely travelled further than the city and then only to our cousins in the country. If we travelled abroad it was to stay with foreign families as part of our education as we reached adulthood, and in my case to complete my medical education in London. My parents took two weeks' holiday a year, to Lucan, Galway, Kerry or Wexford. We were reasonably housed but could have been better clothed to avoid the prevailing chilblains and to reduce our dependence on heating. We were adequately fed although our tastes were simple and eating habits were more disciplined then. The obesity syndrome was to wait many more years. We had the grounds to grow some of our own food and fruit, and to provide eggs for the family and a few other households in the area. We had a large galvanised water butt for use in the garden and greenhouse. Washing dried on the line outside or, when it rained, in the kitchen. Our garden was teeming with insects, bees and butterflies in the summer and with birds at all seasons. We had access to the local library, saw little crime and were at least as happy as an equivalent family today and probably more secure.

As children, we caused no damage to the environment. Indoor games and self-entertainment, added to the girls' activities in designing, creating and repairing clothes, kept us busy, and outdoor games and hobbies were enjoyed and sometimes shared with neighbours and cousins. The emphasis was still on non-elitist sport and regular physical activity. Scouting for the boys was invaluable in terms of occupation, education and training. There was no accumulation of toys and plastic in the house – it was long before the plastic era and the heavy pressure on parents and friends to provide the huge variety of plastic toys so attractive to the young today.

Above all when I was young there was little waste and no evidence of the current pollution of the environment or of unwelcome incinerators. The only possible damage to the environment we might have wrought was the high birth rate, the gradual elimination of the contagious epidemic diseases which had so drastically controlled population in the past and the huge decline in infant mortality. These factors were to contribute to the emerging rapid increase in world population.

Why do we not return to such community existence and thus eliminate the worst elements of globalisation that must inevitably lead to disaster for the world and for humanity? And look at the advantages which we have over and above my family of seventy-five years ago. The dramatic progress of communication by internet, radio and television; the technical advances in food production and product manufacture; the advances in clothing and insulation of houses and offices, the remarkable advances in bike technology and equipment (see the bikers and their families on the Ile de Ré in France!) and in public transportation; the great improvement in general health thanks to prevention, public education and advances in medicine; the great advances in education for the masses and, finally, the inspirational resources of the human mind; and all this without causing damage to the good earth or its inhabitants. We will continue to need energy to provide essential services, but we surely could have access to and utilise solar power more widely and, perhaps to a lesser degree, wind and water energy and energy from the earth's core. A worldwide change from a meat to a vegetable agricultural economy would provide enough food to cater for an inflated human population.

As I write this, I read for the first time the encyclical referring to the environment issued by Pope Benedict XVI. I would have thought it was God's intention that the Church should be responsible for the welfare of Creation as well as the welfare of our souls. But the Church has ignored its role in espousing the welfare of nature and future generations through its neglect of the environment and its encouragement of a disastrous policy supporting an increase in the human population, which is incompatible with the wellbeing of the planet. The Pope needs to do much more to overcome the threat to future generations than publish the bland reference to the environment which is referred to in the recent encyclical. There is worldwide denial about our role in endangering humanity and our natural surroundings. Denial may be based on ignorance, but in many cases we do not wish to know.

The politicians cannot help, for they are subservient to the commercial world, the energy and defence industries, the huge vested interests that control the globalised world, not to mention an electorate obsessed with a culture of wealth, acquisition and the neglect of our natural surroundings upon which we depend for our lives. Political ineptitude is inevitable and it is surely unreal that our Green Party is in government and espousing the building of an expensive and environmentally disastrous incinerator instead of doing all in their power to reduce waste in every form. No Green Party member should be a member of any western government while the politicians are so ineffective.

We need a powerful mass movement by the people to overcome the ineptitude of our politicians and the failure of religious leadership if we are to face the real threat to our planet and future generations. Without a powerful mass movement we will face Nemesis, the Greek concept of retribution, when we ignore our dependence on our natural surroundings. Sadly, Ireland, once described as 'the land of saints and scholars', is among the worst nations in the world in terms of environmental abuse.

'The Peace of Wild Things' by Wendell Berry

When despair for the world grows in me
And I wake in the night at the least sound
In fear of what my life and my children's lives may be,
I go and lie down where the wood drake
Rests in his beauty on the water, and the great heron feeds.
I come into the peace of wild things
Who do not tax their lives with forethought
Of grief. I come into the presence of still water.
And I feel above me the day-blind stars
Waiting with their light. For a time
I rest in the grace of the world, and am free.

Books by Risteárd Mulcahy

Prevention of Coronary Disease (1978)

Beat Heart Disease (1979)

The Long-term Care of the Coronary Patient (1990)

Heart Attack and Lifestyle (1990)

For Love of Trees (1996)

Richard Mulcahy (1886-1971): A Family Memoir (1999)

Improving with Age: What Exercise Can Do for You (2004)

Is the Health Service for Healing? A Doctor's Defence of Medicine's Samaritan Role (2006)

My Father, the General: Richard Mulcahy and the Military History of the Revolution (2009)